ON THE SHOULDERS
OF WOMEN

ON THE SHOULDERS OF WOMEN

The Feminization of Psychotherapy

Ilene J. Philipson

GUILFORD PRESS

New York   London

Printed in the United States of America

This book is printed on acid-free paper.

Last digit is print number: 9 8 7 6 5 4 3 2 1

Library of Congress Cataloging-in-Publication Data

Philipson, Ilene J.
    On the shoulders of women : the feminization of psychotherapy /
Ilene J. Philipson.
        p.   cm.
    Revision of the author's doctoral dissertation at the Wright
Institute.
    Includes bibliographical references and index.
    ISBN 0–89862–017–1
    1. Women psychotherapists—United States—Social conditions.
    2. Psychotherapy—Practice—United States.   3. Sexual division of
labor—United States.   I. Title.
    [DNLM   1. Psychotherapy.   2. Women.   3. Women's Rights.
WM 420   P555o   1993]
RC480.5.P478   1993
616.89'14'082—dc20
DNLM/DLC
for Library of Congress   93-25404
                                                              CIP

Acknowledgments

This book was originally intended as a small, empirical study, and I have only Saul Siegel to thank for talking some well needed sense into me to make it into something longer, more historical, and more speculative. I am grateful to him, Nancy Chodorow, and Anne Bernstein for their comments on the first draft of the manuscript, a doctoral dissertation at the Wright Institute.

For turning the manuscript into the present book, I have relied on many people's comments, time, support, and information. First, I would like to acknowledge the Beatrice M. Bain Research Group at the University of California, Berkeley campus for sponsoring me as an affiliated scholar throughout the research and writing of this book. The scholar meetings were extremely useful, cross-disciplinary study groups that allowed me to present my ideas to women from both the humanities and social sciences. The comments and support of Carla Golden and Roberta Hamilton from the Bain Group were particularly valuable. Second, my "progressive therapists" study group (we've had trouble coming up with a name for ourselves) discussed my ideas on a number of occasions and each time offered fresh perspectives and criticisms that I hope are reflected throughout the book. In particular I wish to thank Andrea Aidells, Diane Ehrensaft, Ron Elson, Anne Bernstein, and Barbara Haber. And it is to Anne and Barbara that parts of this book owe a specific debt. Anne was a generous teacher in the field of family therapy; Chapter 4 could not have been written without her help (any errors or misinterpretations are mine alone). Barbara's influence pervades the book. Our conversations about the current state of psychotherapy practice, what it means for women practitioners, and how it affects these practitioners' sense of themselves always provoked me to think more and harder about the matter at hand. While I know she does not agree with all of my analyses and assessments, I hope she discerns her significant contribution to my thinking.

Jeffrey Escoffier allowed me to see how to transform a somewhat clunky, academic dissertation into a more smoothly flowing book. For over a decade he has been critiquing my work, taking whatever ideas I come up with and turning them back to me with twists, applications, and meanings that I could never envision on my own. While he has lent his editorial wizardry to virtually everything I have published, even more importantly, he remains an intellectual mentor, an unceasing explorer of the landscape of ideas, who often takes me along for the ride.

Many others have contributed in big and small ways, from reading chapters to granting me formal interviews to providing important pieces of information or insight. I would like to thank Greg Alter, Colin Bell, Jessica Benjamin, Elliott Currie, Florence Denmark, Sue Elkind, Anthea Fursland, Christina Halsey, Otto Kernberg, Elizabeth Knoll, Jessica Kohout, Chris Lehmann, Jean Baker Miller, Kitty Moore, Andrea Morrison, Lynn O'Connor, Peggy Papp, Rachael Peltz, Ethel Person, David Pingitore, David Robishone, Olga Silverstein, and Robert Wallerstein. I would also like to thank Karen Hansen for sponsoring a talk based on my research at the Bunting Institute at Radcliffe College, and Roberta Hamilton for sponsoring one at Queen's University in Kingston, Ontario. I am also grateful to the editors of *Tikkun* magazine and *Sociological Practice Review* for publishing two articles of mine which helped in the development of Chapters 1 and 6 of this book.

Michael Goldhaber served as on-the-spot editorial consultant, constant emotional support, and ceaseless creator of snappy titles and subtitles. I am so very grateful to him. Lastly, Rudy and Amos were tireless companions throughout the writing of the entire book; they literally were always at my side. Their patience, constancy, and unspoken love repeatedly showed me how trivial mere words can often be.

Contents

ON THE SHOULDERS
OF WOMEN

CHAPTER 1

Introduction

With little fanfare or professional acknowledgment, a fundamental transformation is taking place in the field of psychotherapy: It is becoming a women's occupation. Fewer men
and increasing numbers of women are entering the field,
making the prototypical "shrink" a woman.

Feminization represents a significant alteration of the
field. Two professional categories of psychotherapists—clinical social workers and marriage and family counselors
(master's level clinical psychologists)—have always belonged
to women (with at least 70% of the practitioners female).[1] A
third category, psychiatry, is moving away from the practice
of psychotherapy entirely. Increasingly unable to compete
with the typically lower fees of psychologists and social workers, psychiatry as a profession is turning its back on psychotherapy altogether and focusing on biological psychiatry
(Goleman, 1990). Yet even in this "remedicalized" field, feminization is gradually occurring. In 1979, women represented
31.5% of all psychiatric residents, and by 1989, 41%. The
fourth and final category, however, has witnessed a truly
remarkable rise in the percentage of practitioners who are
female. In 1976, 31.1% of all recipients of Ph.D.'s in clinical
psychology in the United States were women, but by 1990,
they made up over 58% (Kohout, 1991). This contrasts markedly with the fact that since the mid-1980s, men's receipt of

---

[1]According to Strober and Arnold (1987), "an occupation can be termed
female dominated or female intensive if 60% or more of the workers in
that occupation were female" (p. 108).

1

doctorates in clinical psychology has decreased by an average of almost 2% annually (Ostertag & McNamara, 1991, p. 353).

I believe that these twin phenomena of women's rise in participation and men's decline must be viewed in larger context. As I hope to demonstrate throughout this book, the feminization of psychotherapy can only be understood through its complex interconnection with both the current crisis in the practice of psychotherapy and the gender segregation of work that pervades our society in general.

The Crisis in Psychotherapy

There should be little question today that the practice of psychotherapy is in tumult. Professional publications tell of a "mental health care revolution" in which the state increasingly abdicates responsibility for funding services, insurance carriers deem psychological treatment an unnnecessary luxury, and the independent practitioner is threatened with occupational extinction (see Zimet, 1989).

Over the course of the past decade, federal, state, and local monies for virtually every form of mental health service have been decisively reduced. Not only for the poor but also for much of the working class, there are simply no affordable mental health services available. Even in the case of drug addiction, a problem that is presumably of the highest priority in our society, clients often have to wait months for any form of treatment, due to understaffed clinics and huge waiting lists. Only when an individual becomes dangerous—suicidal or homicidal—can the few remnants of the community mental health system be quickly brought to bear. Even then, however, the system offers at best a few days of hospitalization, antipsychotic or antidepressant medication, and release back into the community with little more than a prescription and an appointment with a psychiatrist in a month or two to monitor the medication's effects.

That mental illness contributes significantly to mounting homelessness, some violent crime, and drug and alcohol addiction has yet to galvanize politicians into supporting mental health services. Instead, our tolerance for bizarre, confrontational, and violent behavior on our streets and in public places is simply forced to expand. As Matthew Dumont, a pioneer of the early community mental health movement, has noted, we are "returning to the era before Dorothea Dix" (quoted in Wylie, 1992b, p. 13).

Although the state supports the use of psychoactive drugs for the treatment of psychological problems, it is clear that it has virtually abandoned any commitment to or interest in psychotherapy. Clearly the idea of funding a process that may take weeks, months, or years is unpalatable when many local governments teeter on financial collapse and when the omnipresent quick fix of drug therapy is advertised as a cost-saving alternative. Yet it is not only those who look to the state for help who are affected by this narrowing vision. As health care costs in general have skyrocketed, employers and insurance carriers have progressively cut back on reimbursements to the private practitioners who minister to the working and middle classes. According to the U.S. Bureau of Labor Statistics, only 21% of large U.S. companies offered the same level of mental health benefits in 1989 as they did in 1980 (Garrison, 1991, p. 1).

"Managed health care"—the health maintenance organization (HMO) or preferred provider organization (PPO)—is the means by which increasing numbers of people are obtaining health services. These organizations also view psychotherapy as a treatment they can ill afford to support. Typically they allow their subscribers three to six visits with a psychotherapist, in rare instances as many as twenty, but not more. If after 1 to 4 months of treatment a psychological problem is not resolved, there is no appeal, no further help. While this sort of stance toward physical illness would be incomprehensible, it has become routine in the treatment of psychic disorder.

Ironically, however, as public and private funding sources for psychotherapy services have radically declined, the number of people becoming psychotherapists has dramatically increased. In the decade between 1975 and 1985, the number of psychiatrists increased by 46%; the number of clinical psychologists (Ph.D.'s) by 80%; the number of social workers by 140%, and the number of marriage and family counselors (master's level clinical psychologists) by an astounding 367% (Robiner, 1991, p. 428). Quite simply, graduate programs are turning out huge numbers of clinicians at a time when support for psychotherapy is dwindling in all sectors of society.

It is in this context that psychotherapy as an occupation is being feminized. Due both to greater numbers of women and fewer numbers of men entering psychotherapy training programs, clinical practice is moving toward becoming a professional world without men. Conventional wisdom gleaned from other fields that have feminized indicates that when men abandon an occupational category, the field becomes less remunerative and lower in status. There seems to be little reason to believe that psychotherapy will differ from this pattern, particularly given ever-increasing competition within the field, the shrinking job market, and a growing belief within psychiatry—and perhaps among the public in general—that drugs offer a better chance for cure than talking.

If the feminization of psychotherapy were only a professional issue, however, the topic probably could be addressed sufficiently within the confines of professional journals and forums. But feminization does not merely alter the gender of the field's typical practitioner. It affects the theories that guide that practitioner's work within the consulting room, her views of psychopathology and of human development. In fact, feminization can be seen as integral to the transformation in the reigning paradigms that govern the very techniques and goals of psychotherapeutic practice, as I hope to illuminate in this book.

But the implications of feminization go even further, transcending the boundaries of clinical theory and practice altogether. The gender transformation in the field of psychotherapy—an institution in crisis and increasingly populated by women practitioners—mirrors changes in the contemporary family—an institution in crisis and increasingly populated by mothers parenting alone. I believe that the feminization of psychotherapy reflects larger changes regarding the relative responsibility of men and women in society to provide intimacy, care, and what sociologist Arlie Hochschild (1983) has called "emotion work." Men's declining involvement in psychotherapy—much like many men's declining involvement in families—reinforces the widely held belief that it is women and not men who are responsible for tending to and ameliorating our emotional pain and psychological problems. Because our society denigrates this kind of emotion work, women therapists—just as women in families—are finding it increasingly difficult to be supported economically for the work they do.

This is not to say, however, that for many women the experience of becoming a psychotherapist has not resulted in a greater sense of self-esteem and personal gratification. But increased competition and downturns in the field due to cutbacks in public and private funding are stymieing many women's desire to fulfill their professional goals. With fewer jobs available, they open private practices and compete with each other to find clients who can pay out of pocket. For those who do find salaried positions, their work is often doing "McTherapy," seeing more than 36 clients a week under the auspices of HMOs or PPOs, which have become the fast-food franchises of mental health care. These therapists practice psychotherapy with almost no autonomy or control over the work process, and they often are unable to offer long-lasting help in the three to six sessions each client is allotted.

Since the theories that underlie the practice of psychotherapy typically eschew social explanations of human unhappiness, therapists are only too ready to see themselves as the ultimate source of any professional problems they may have. Many women new to the field see their work difficulties as personal and idiosyncratic, results of their own psychological problems or defects as clinicians. If they turn to their own therapists for understanding, they often hear the interpretations frequently applied to women who face problems with work: fear of success, guilt over competence, desire to fail, anxiety over being more successful than one's parents. Virtually no one in the field speaks of the implications of years of cutbacks in mental health funding on psychotherapists themselves or of the proliferation of freestanding professional schools that charge their students tens of thousands of dollars in tuition and then graduate them into a market that cannot adequately remunerate them for their services, nor provide employment commensurate with their abilities and training. These women become healers who are not allowed to heal, professionals who want to help others in a world that accords little recognition and decreasing remuneration to emotion work and caregiving of all kinds.

The fate of psychotherapy and its increasingly female body of practitioners speaks to our society's devaluation of caregiving and women's identification with this devalued arena of life. As the well-being of children—both within families and schools[2]—the elderly, animals,[3] the mentally ill, and the emotionally injured rests increasingly on women's shoulders' alone, the public and private sectors withdraw support and observe from a distance the single mother, the inner-city female school teacher, the woman psychotherapist as she attempts to work under increasingly adverse circumstances. What is occurring in the field of psychotherapy reveals a disturbing trend that seems to haunt our social landscape.

I decided to undertake this study after beginning graduate school in clinical psychology. Having received a doctorate in sociology 7 years earlier, I was startled to realize that I now had entered what appeared to be an all-women's field. As I sat in classes and undertook clinical internships in which 80% to 90% of the students and interns were women, I thought back to the mid-1970s when I entered graduate school in sociology and many of my friends were becoming clinical psychologists. At that time, most of the clinical psychology programs with which I was familiar appeared to have

---

[2]"The National Education Association found that the percentage of men teaching in elementary schools has fallen to the lowest point in a quarter-century. . . . In 1991, only 12% of kindergarten to sixth-grade teachers were male, down from 13.8% in 1986 and 17.7% in 1981" ("Survey Finds Fewer Men," 1992).

[3]This refers to the fact that veterinary medicine has recently undergone a process of feminization.

equal numbers of women and men, much like the sociology program in which I was enrolled. Something clearly had occurred in the intervening decade, transforming the gender composition of the profession. But no one seemed to acknowledge this transformation, let alone attempt to account for it.

As my training took me to more and more clinical settings, I began to notice a pattern: a largely female staff of therapists with male or male and female supervisors and clinical directors. In the public sector, most directors were fighting battles to keep their agencies alive through the use of unpaid psychology interns like myself and through staff cutbacks. Often a sense of doom or desperation pervaded the work setting as smaller staffs and/or less experienced therapists attempted to confront the ravages of drug and alcohol addiction, AIDS, personality disorders, economic dislocation, child sexual abuse, family disintegration, and the ordinary unhappiness that psychotherapists from Sigmund Freud on have considered their mainstay. At one family services agency in a wealthy suburb, the director kept his clinic going by paying interns nothing and his staff therapists—some with 20 years of experience or more—$16 an hour. If a client cancelled or did not appear for an appointment, the therapist received nothing. At a community crisis clinic in a large metropolitan area that ministers to the homeless, the homicidal, the suicidal, the psychotic, and the severely addicted, on any single shift one paid therapist supervised the work of three to ten unpaid graduate students who did all the direct patient care. In the outpatient psychotherapy department of a large urban hospital, the staff consisted of a quarter-time director, a half-time intake worker, and a full-time receptionist and bookkeeper. All the clinicians were unpaid interns. In a private, for-profit, managed care agency, money abounded, but clinicians were closely monitored to see that their average number of sessions per client did not exceed three. Working full time, a clinician could carry a caseload of 50, given that many clients were encouraged not to attend therapy more than twice a month. The language of cost containment and profitability could be heard more readily than the words patient care.

What all of these diverse settings had in common was a dearth of men. The ratio of female to male therapists ranged anywhere from three to one, to ten to one. Male interns were in extremely short supply, and it was commonly acknowledged that virtually any male applicant for an internship position would be considered, whereas female applicants were in superabundance and therefore had to avidly compete with each other. While men were visible as clinical supervisors and agency directors, it fell to the woman practitioner to handle the suicidal or addicted client, to explain why a client could not see her for more than three sessions, to receive no compensation when her scheduled client failed to appear for his or her appointment.

In an attempt to support themselves upon graduation and begin paying back the student loans they had acquired as graduate students, and in order to practice their profession, many of the clinical psychologists with whom I graduated attempted to set up part-time private practices. But a decline in third-party payments, ever-growing competition among practitioners, and a nationwide recession conspired to make the feasibility of such undertaking extremely problematic. With each private practitioner seeing ten or fewer clients for fees that covered only rent, malpractice insurance, and consultation fees, very few were able to support themselves, and many turned to part-time work in nonpsychotherapy-related jobs or in agencies that hired contract workers for $15 to $20 an hour. Some found jobs in managed care administration, in which they had no direct patient contact and were paid less than their colleagues who did contract work.

Both the rapidly deteriorating environment for mental health services and feminization envelop the world of psychotherapy. Yet almost no one I encountered as a graduate student and intern, or whom I meet today in my current role as a practicing psychotherapist, seeks to discuss these issues. Feminization seems to be taken for granted, while the crisis in mental health care is often understood in terms of the therapist's own difficulties in her private practice, clinic, or un- or underemployment. It is her idiosyncratic problem to be addressed through improved marketing skills, innovative fundraising for her agency, or self-improvement as a thera-pist. As a sociologist I am bewildered by the narrowness of this vision and alarmed by the self-blame that it entails.

This book is an attempt, then, to address my bewilder-ment and expand the narrow vision that currently prevents a psychotherapist from looking beyond the confines of her own consulting room and perhaps her own feelings of self-blame. It is an effort to understand the reasons for and the consequences of the feminization of psychotherapy. And it is one means of trying to understand what is happening to our national priorities, our collective sense of social responsibil-ity, and our deeply gendered notions of who carries out those responsibilities and under what conditions.

The Feminization of Work

While the crisis enveloping the practice of psychotherapy forms one backdrop for the feminization of the field, another is the pervasive segregation of the world of work along gen-der lines and the current feminization of many factions of the labor force (Jenson, Hagen, & Eddy, 1988). Occupational sex segregation, or the sexual division of labor, is a cross-cultural and historically enduring social phenomenon. What *types* of work are deemed male or female, however, differ significantly among cultures and can vary over time in any one society. While the United States' occupational structure has been seg-regated by gender throughout its history, sex typing of spe-cific kinds of work and job categories has changed to varying degrees over the course of the historical record.

Sex segregation within the labor market has been more resistant to change than segregation based on any other demographic category, including race. Even though a num-ber of job categories have changed in their gender composi-tion since World War II, overall labor market segregation by sex has remained remarkably stable over time. About two thirds of American men and women would have to change occupations today in order to achieve equal gender distribu-tion across occupations, a figure that was the same in 1900

(Strober & Arnold, 1987, p. 108). Women remain concentrated in a small number of jobs that have been labeled women's work since the turn of the century or before. Nursing, teaching, clerical work, and routinized, unskilled assembly line work remain bastions of female employment. In 1985 over two thirds of the women in the U.S. civilian labor force worked in occupations that were 70% or more female (Jacobs, 1989, p. 1).

Even when women and men share an occupation, they typically do jobs within the occupation that are dissimiliar. In their study of 11 occupations that are currently in the process of being transformed from predominantly male to predominantly female in composition, Reskin and Roos found that men and women were concentrated in different jobs in every case, even though they had the same occupational title. Men held the most desirable jobs, while women were disproportionately relegated to jobs having lower status, less desirable work settings, lower pay, and part-time rather than full-time employment. Thus, despite the feminizing process, men held onto the better jobs within the occupational classification that was undergoing gender recomposition (Reskin & Roos, 1990, p. 72).

This sort of sex segregation within occupations is true not only for blue-collar and white-collar work but for professional work as well. The examples of library science, public school teaching, and law are illustrative.

At present about 82% of all librarians are female. Even though women have constituted the majority of practitioners in this occupational category virtually since its inception, except when discussing numerical representation alone, it would be deceptive to characterize library science as a female-dominated field. Librarianship may be a feminized profession but it is controlled by men. Although women have constituted about 80% of the American Library Association (ALA) since the turn of the century, 75% of the presidents of the ALA have been men. Salary surveys of librarians have consistently shown that male librarians receive higher salaries for almost all job-level categories within the profession. And among medical librarians, to cite but one specialty, men occupy most top-level management positions, while women are clustered at low- and mid-management levels, again despite their numerical domination of the field (Kenkel, 1991, pp. 11–12).

In the case of public school teaching, women constitute 83.5% of the elementary school teachers but only 16.9% of the elementary school principals. Fifty percent of secondary school teachers are women, but a mere 3.5% of the principals are women. Of all public school personnel 66% are women, but only 3% of the school superintendents are women (Kenkel, 1991, p. 12).

Unlike library science or teaching, law has traditionally both been numerically dominated and controlled by men. Yet women increasingly are entering the field. In 1951 women represented only 2.5% of the legal profession, whereas in 1985 they made up 13.1% of the legal work force. By the early 1980s women constituted one third of those accepted to law school, and by the early 1990s in many law schools across the country this percentage had increased to one half.

Despite these increases, what kinds of law women practice and where they work perpetuates job-level segregation of the legal profession. Women tend to cluster in lower-status practices, such as those dealing with divorce, juvenile, and welfare cases, while rarely engaging in the higher-status specialties, such as tax law and corporate litigation (Touhey, 1974, p. 86). They also are overrepresented in legal clinics, where work is routinized and opportunities for advancement are few (Reskin & Roos, 1990, p. 72).

However, within the overall context of our deeply gendered world of work, women have moved into various traditional male preserves at a steady clip since the 1970s. Historically, women have entered occupations when they have been permitted to do so. Once explicit or implicit barriers to women's participation are abandoned, women seek admission, often in overwhelming numbers. Two earlier examples of the rapid entry of women into fields from which they had been previously barred are clerical work in the 19th century and welding and coal mining during World War II (Reskin & Hartmann, 1986, p. 77; Williams, 1989).

Within this rubric there are various general characteristics that attract women to jobs. The compatibility with child care and domestic concerns is often cited as primary. Related to this is the desire for work that is not dangerous, that is close to home, that can be readily interrupted, and that offers flexible hours (Reskin & Hartmann, 1986, p. 7). These requirements have become particularly salient given the changing composition of the female labor force. While earlier in the century the typical working woman was single without children, today she is just as likely to be married and a mother. As of 1986, 51% of women with children younger than age 3 were employed. And it is married or divorced women between the ages of 30 and 44 who have experienced one of the sharpest rises in their labor force participation within the last two decades.

Since the 1970s a number of occupations have changed from being largely male occupations to being largely female ones. Insurance adjuster and examiner, real estate agent, book editor, bartender, and baker are among the jobs that have undergone this transformation. While each occupation has some unique factors that lead to and result from the feminizing process, there are a number of general characteristics that accompany occupational gender transposition.

When work becomes feminized the chief implications are that it becomes less remunerative and lower status. Quite simply, as an occupation grows in its percentage of female workers, its wages decline proportionately. Thus both women *and men* in female-dominated occupations experience lower pay (Reskin & Hartmann, 1986, p. 10). According to a report of the National Research Council's Committee on Occupational Classification and Analysis, the overall earning differential between women and men in American society—women earn about 68¢ for every $1 men make—can be attributed to the low wages women earn in predominantly female occupations (Reskin & Hartmann, 1986, p. 10).

The perceived status of an occupation also declines when feminization occurs. As Everett Hughes long ago asserted, an occupation comes to be defined by the secondary characteristics of those who occupy the role (cited in Bourne & Wikler,

1982). In a study conducted by John Touhey (1974), significant differences in the prestige and desirability of a profession were found to exist when a profession was characterized as undergoing feminization. College students rated the occupations architect, college professor, lawyer, physician, and scientist significantly lower in prestige and desirability when they were told that the proportion of female practitioners was increasing in these professions. On semantic differential scales, the students rated professions in the process of feminization to be more passive than active, more insecure than secure, more unsuccessful than successful, and more useless than useful. These findings did not differ according to the sex of the subject who did the rating.

In a similar but more recent study, Jerry Jacobs (1989) found that men were rated higher on a prestige scale in male-dominated occupations, while women were rated higher in female-dominated occupations. He concluded from this that "incumbency in sex-atypical occupational roles is associated with a 'prestige penalty.' These data can be viewed as suggesting that there is a cost to sex-role deviance" (p. 34).

Further, in a qualitative study of women in the Marine Corps and men in nursing, Christine Williams (1989) found that men avoided female-dominated jobs not only because of their lower pay but due to their association with "'nonmasculine' character traits—and most men do not want to be considered nonmasculine" (p. 141). Of the male nurses she interviewed, many argued that they had not entered nursing "freely" but as a result of their previous job experience or their perception of having only limited work opportunities open to them.

> In fact, the men I interviewed told me that nursing was probably the last occupation they would have considered in their youth; its close association as a women's profession is a formidable barrier to any male otherwise inclined to do this type of work. To encourage more men in nursing, they argued, the first order of business should be to change this feminine connotation. One man even recommended changing the name of the profession because "nursing semantically denotes women—breastfeeding. [It's] considered a female profession, and males

in the field [are believed to] have feminine characteristics."
As long as nursing is defined as "women's work," men will
simply *not want to* engage in it. (pp. 140–141)

The Reasons for Feminization

Given the effect of lower remuneration, status, and desirability, why do occupations become feminized? While there
appear to be a number of responses to this question, the
answer seems to originate in three potentially related but distinct directions. First, when an occupation begins to decline
in earnings, benefits, prestige, job security, autonomy, or
chances for advancement relative to comparable occupations,
men tend to move out. As more men begin to view a declining occupation as "on the skids," the doors are open for
women to replace the men who have vacated the jobs or who
are simply not entering them as much as they once did
(Reskin & Roos, 1990, p. 47). Second, if an occupation experiences rapid growth to the point of creating a shortfall of
male workers, women may be enlisted into the ranks. This
would typically be the case when education, special training,
or some form of credentialing delimits the available pool of
men, and employers are forced to look to women. Third, the
growth of a female clientele for any occupation can prompt
employers to hire women in order to better serve customers.
"A highly sex-differentiated society creates a demand for
workers (such as coaches, counselors, and prison guards) who
are the same sex as their occupational role partners" (Reskin
& Roos, 1990, p. 104). A fourth, historically specific reason
that may account for the beginning of the feminizing process
is the recent antidiscrimination regulations and litigation that
have made it illegal to give men preference in job hiring,
wages, and promotion.

While these reasons account for the inception of the
move toward feminization, they do not fully describe how
some occupations become fully feminized. When an occupation is transformed in its composition from being predominantly male to predominantly female (or vice versa), "reseg-

regation" has taken place. Therefore, it is important to see change in an occupation's gender composition as a process. What may appear to be integration of women and men at a single point in history, may turn out to be resegregation at a later point in time (Reskin & Roos, 1990, p. 72). In this regard economists often refer to the parallels between neighborhood racial resegregation and occupational gender resegregation (Reskin & Roos, 1990, p. 314; Strober & Arnold, 1987, pp. 116–117). Strober and Arnold (1987) suggest that there exists a "tipping point" of female employment in a specific occupation, beyond which men begin "to move rapidly out of the occupation, fearing that the occupation would become female and hence reduced in both status and pay" (p. 117). While such a tipping point cannot be predicted for any one occupation, it is determined in part by the specifics of the occupation and the historical period in which resegregation occurs.

Since the latter half of the 19th century, the historical record is replete with examples of occupations that have undergone feminization. By looking at some of these, it may be possible to gain a better understanding of the tenets set forth above, and also to find specific historical material that may inform our investigation of the feminization of psychotherapy.

Clerical work (along with public school teaching) is one of the earliest examples of an occupation that changed from being predominantly male to predominantly female. In 1870, 4% of stenographers and typists were women. Ten years later, women accounted for 40% of these occupations, and in 1900, 77%. By 1930, 95% of all typists and stenographers were women, a statistic that has remained relatively constant since that time.

This startling transformation can be ascribed to a number of factors: the vast expansion of clerical work following the Civil War; the introduction of the typewriter, and the decline in autonomy and chances for advancement among clerical workers.

According to historian Margery Davies (1982), the growth and consolidation of business and industry after the

Civil War effected a sharp increase in the amount of correspondence and record keeping required (p. 55). This increase led employers to institute a far more hierarchical division of labor, creating specialized jobs such as filing, shipping, and billing clerks, where formerly such tasks were performed by a single person who more resembled a professional manager than today's clerical worker. During the 1870s and 1880s the typewriter was first marketed on a wide basis. Remington Company, which developed the typewriter, opened typewriting schools in large cities and established employment bureaus attached to them in order to teach typewriting and facilitate the employment of typists. The vast majority of students were women. Because a typist had to "be a good speller, a good grammarian and have the correct knowledge of the use of capitals and the rules of punctuation," only people with the requisite educational skills were appropriate students (cited in Rothman, 1978, p. 48). This ruled out the blue-collar male worker. And neither the skilled male worker nor the middle-class man with a high school education would be attracted to a typist job, which did not pay as well as either the skilled trades or most forms of white-collar or professional employment. "Recognizing that men were either ineligible or uninterested, the company then turned to women, to the large pool of female high school graduates" (Rothman, 1978, p. 49).

As clerical work became increasingly feminized, wages declined relative to jobs in manufacturing. Chances for promotion became negligible as the routine tasks involved in typing and stenography could not readily translate into any management position. And any autonomy and control over the work process that had existed prior to the introduction of the typewriter and the hierarchical reorganization of clerical labor disappeared as employers hired more and more women whom they believed to be "uniquely suited to boring, menial tasks where qualities of leadership or independence were totally unnecessary" (Davies, 1982, p. 174). Within 30 years the fundamental nature of clerical work had changed, and so had the gender of its practitioners.

We return in the end to the significance of the feminization of the clerical labor force. It meant that the degradation of clerical work and the proletarianization of the office workers was diguised. . . . [T]he decline in their position relative to their nineteenth-century predecessors' was masked. . . . The nineteenth-century clerk had not turned into a proletarian; he had merely turned into a woman. (Davies, 1982, pp. 174–175)

The example of bank telling is another occupation that experienced rapid feminization. In a period of 45 years, between 1935 and 1980, it went from being virtually all male to 91% female.

During World War I women were recruited to become bank tellers, but once the war ended were quickly replaced by men. During the period between the two wars, bank telling was reorganized somewhat along the lines of "deskilling," in which complex jobs are broken down into simpler tasks. Within the bank structure, a greater hierarchy of jobs was created and with this an accompanying pay hierarchy. Because of these changes, women entered the field at increasing rates. They were more willing to work for lower wages and were viewed by employers as appropriate for work assignments at the lower ends of the job hierarchy. These jobs demanded little responsibility for the money handled, necessitated minimal supervision, and offered virtually no autonomy or control over the work performed. Due to these developments, by the beginning of World War II, women constituted 37% of the bank telling occupation.

With World War II, due to the need to replace male employees who had been recruited by the armed forces, employers were forced to streamline the training process for tellers. From 5 years of on-the-job training, teller training was reduced to 6 weeks of full-time study and 1 month on the job. But it was not only training that changed during the war. Before the late 1930s and early 1940s banks primarily served corporations and wealthy individuals. Few people actually held checking accounts. In order to have more access to funds during the Depression and war years, banks began offering new services to larger segments of the population. They introduced "economy checking accounts" with no minimum balance requirements and minimal monthly charges to maintain checking accounts. They also made installment loans for consumer purchases, real estate, and small business investments available to the public, and they began accepting telephone and utility payments.

In the postwar economic boom, the public responded enthusiastically to these services. Between 1939 and 1952, the number of checking accounts in the United States increased from 27 million to 47.1 million. Banks, in turn, expanded their number of branches in urban and suburban settings and instituted innovations such as sidewalk tellers and drive-in windows. As a consequence, the overall number of bank employees increased during this period, as did the proportion of those employees who were tellers.

With this "shift from class to mass banking," the status of bank telling declined, and with it, its wages relative to similar occupations, and ultimately, its attractiveness to male employees, who could find comparable jobs elsewhere for higher pay and higher status. The image of the job and its association with a lower class of customer probably had more to do with the occupation's decline than any change in the job's tasks (Strober & Arnold, 1987, p. 132). Thus, the process of "declassing" enabled female employees to hold on to their teller jobs following World War II. Men did not reclaim these jobs despite the fact that employers offered bank teller training classes for returning male veterans. By 1950, women filled almost half of all bank telling positions. For the next 30 years "customers and services became much more common and less elite," and women continued to grow in their numerical domination of the bank telling occupation (Strober & Arnold, 1987, p. 132). In 1960, 69% of all bank tellers were women; by 1970, 86%, and by 1980, 91%.

Therefore, while deskilling allowed for the entry of women into the field in the period between the two wars, it appears that declassing accounted for the feminization of bank telling after World War II. That is, what caused the occupation to "tip" into being a female field was the status change that resulted from declassing, that is, the shift from class to mass banking.

As a final example, the recent transformation of book editing from a male to female profession highlights some further characteristics of feminization. Until quite recently, book editing was considered a "gentleman's profession." Due to its association with high culture, intellectuality, and the arts, its low pay and detachment from the world of commerce, book editing attracted men from the upper classes and Ivy League schools. In the first 60 years of the 20th century, even though men overwhelmingly dominated the profession, women held a number of jobs. They were concentrated in children's publishing, and, to a lesser degree, mass-market paperback publishing, and they held positions that bridged clerical work and editorial work, such as copyediting, editorial assistance, and manuscript reading.

In the 1960s, however, this picture began to change. With rising personal income, educational levels, and federal investments in public education, people began buying books in record numbers. In response to this growth in readership, the already existing publishing houses expanded their lists, while at least 300 new publishers emerged between 1967 and 1978. Both title output and sales volume showed increases of 50% to 100% between 1959 and 1980 (Reskin, 1990, p. 98).

Due to this kind of growth, in the 1970s nonpublishing firms and conglomerates searching for profitable acquisitions were attracted to the publishing industry. As more and more publishing houses were bought up by these corporations, publishing was rapidly transformed from a "gentleman's profession" to a business concerned primarily with the "bottom line." This commercial focus had a significant impact on book editors' work.

The concern with profit margins and the never-ending search for a "blockbuster" delimited the autonomy of the editor in acquiring books. No longer was he able to acquire a book without the approval of a publishing committee that evaluated potential sales, packaging, marketing, publicity, and subsidiary rights as much as the quality and merit of the

manuscript itself. Increasing control of the publishing industry by conglomerates also threatened editors' job security,
which had often served as the only economic compensation
for the relatively low wages that have characterized editorial
work throughout its history. Mergers, takeovers, and a consistent preoccupation with profits often resulted in the lay-
ing off of book editors throughout the 1970s and 1980s.

These alterations have made book editing less attractive
to men. While the autonomy, status, and job security of the
occupation have declined, its characteristic low wages have
remained the same. Thus higher-paying media jobs (e.g., technical writing for high-tech companies, corporate public relations, film) and graduate school have lured away men who
might have been attracted to the field in earlier times (Reskin,
1990, p. 101).

Just as the character of the publishing world was shifting in the 1970s, women's greater labor force participation
during that decade was creating a larger pool of women available for editorial positions. College educated, skilled in working with words and communication, and typically willing to
take positions for lower salaries than comparably trained men
who enjoyed greater job opportunities, women began entering editorial positions at a far greater rate than men.

In addition to this familiar pattern, however, women also
were sought out as editors due to the feminization of the
audience they served. By the 1970s, women constituted the
majority of the readers and buyers of fiction. Due to the prevailing view that members of any one "minority" group can
serve its own members better than individuals from any other
group (Reskin & Roos, 1990, p. 49), publishers have increasingly recruited female editors to gain greater insight into the
tastes of their growing female audience. The women's movement of the late 1960s and 1970s also led to a rise in the
number of manuscripts submitted to publishing houses by
women intended for an exclusively female audience. This, in
turn, created a demand for editors who could engage with
these authors and their manuscripts in a way that the prototypical book editor of the 1950s and 1960s—a middle-aged
or older man—probably could not. Thus, in addition to

changes in the publishing industry that decreased status, autonomy, and job security while holding salaries at a relatively low level, employers have increasingly hired women to meet the needs of a growing female readership. These changes have resulted in an editorial work force that was about two thirds female by the early 1980s.

These three examples—clerical work, bank telling, and book editing—demonstrate how and why occupations that were formerly male bastions rapidly underwent a process of feminization due to both common and historically unique factors. Each of these occupations went from being completely segregated, to having a brief period of gender integration, to becoming resegregated. While feminization undoubtedly opens up new work possibilities for women, it typically accompanies downturns in an occupational category and acts to then cement these downturns in place, given the devaluation that women's work has in our society.

As the next two chapters demonstrate, the gender transposition of psychotherapy appears to be progressing along lines familiar to those who study the feminization of occupations. But due to the unique work psychotherapists perform, the ramifications of its becoming a women's field are far more multifaceted and wide ranging than for those occupations discussed thus far. Psychotherapy speaks to people's inner core of experience, attempts to understand and heal our deepest wounds, and offers a vision of health, maturity, and personhood. In a quotidian manner, it faces questions of human nature, right and wrong, and the meaning of existence that in previous times were solely the property of philosophy departments and religious institutions. Thus, its feminization, that is, its increasing practice by one gender alone, signals change that I believe transcends any discussion of economics or professional organization. In the remainder of this book, I hope to begin a discussion about what I see as the profound change women's numerical domination of the field portends— not only for psychotherapy but for our society, its priorities and commonly shared ethics and beliefs.

The Triumph of the Therapeutic and Its Decline

In order to understand the causes of the feminization of psychotherapy, it is crucial to see how the field itself has undergone profound transformation. Psychotherapy today bears little resemblance to its namesake in previous decades, and it is in this historical alteration that I believe the prerequisites for feminization find their source. As the field women are inheriting from men differs so markedly from what it was even a decade ago, it is imperative to acknowledge that the very term "psychotherapy" and our associations and attitudes toward it are historically shaped and colored.

If we define psychotherapy as an ongoing, face-to-face encounter between a professional therapist and a client that relies primarily on talking to effect psychological change, it did not exist in anything approaching its present form prior to World War II. When it was practiced before the war it was typically improvised, undertheorized, eclectic, and seen as conjunctional or secondary to other tasks or goals. The two predominant means of treating mental illness—the custodial mental hospital for the psychotic disturbances and psychoanalysis for what was thought of as more neurotic problems—eschewed psychotherapy. In the mental hospital, psychiatrists favored an organic approach to both etiology and treatment. For psychoanalysts, anything less than the "pure gold" of analytic technique (five times a week on the couch focusing on free association and interpretation of resistances) was denigrated, although occasionally improvised for patients unable to tolerate the regressive pulls of analytic treatment.

Psychotherapy was slightly more acknowledged and accepted in two other settings: mental hospitals that adhered to the "new psychiatry" and child guidance clinics. First, the new psychiatry was a novel response to the dominant, 19th century view of severe psychiatric disturbance as a product of exclusively physiological factors. The tenets of the new psychiatry were perhaps best exemplified in the work of Adolf Meyer, who emphasized both social environment and biology to account for mental illness. In contradistinction to the purely organic understanding of psychiatric disturbance that dominated the custodial mental hospital, or insane asylum, Meyer maintained that:

> Just as bacteriology studies the water supply and the air and food of communities, schools, and homes, so we psychopathologists have to study more effectively the atmosphere of the community and must devise safeguards in the localities from which the patients come, and to which they are to return. (quoted in Lubove, 1971, p. 59)

To this end, Meyer stressed the use of both the "psychiatric interview," to gain a detailed understanding of a patient's life history and the events that gave rise to psychological disturbance, and the psychiatric social worker, who could elaborate this history through visits to a patient's family and community. Meyer is generally credited with founding the profession of psychiatric social work, involving the social worker not only in the evaluation of psychiatric patients but also in their treatment through education and support of family members and others in the patient's environment.

Although the new psychiatry was practiced at only a tiny fraction of facilities treating the mentally ill—affecting fewer than 5% of institutionalized mental patients prior to World War II—it made significant inroads at some public hospitals, such as St. Elizabeth's in Washington, D.C., and at a number of private hospitals servicing the wealthy, such as Austen Riggs, Chestnut Lodge, and Menninger. At the latter, the new psychiatry was expanded vastly beyond Meyer's vision into what would come to be called "milieu therapy" in the postwar period (Reisman, 1976, p. 294). As formulated by William Menninger, the mental hospital was no longer a custodial facility, where discrete psychiatric treatments, such as hydrotherapy, insulin shock, or various forms of reeducation were provided, but rather a therapeutic environment, where every member of the staff—from psychiatrist to attendant—participated on some level in treating the patient. Because Menninger insisted that each staff member not only carry out the attending psychiatrist's orders but understand the rationale for those orders, nurses, social workers, and attendants were required to have some minimal grasp of psychoanalytic theory, which was the prevailing paradigm at Menninger.

The second institutional precursor in the development of the field of psychotherapy was the child guidance clinic. The National Committee for Mental Hygiene in conjunction with the Commonwealth Fund established child guidance clinics throughout the United States in the 1920s. Dedicated to the overarching belief in "preventative mental hygiene," these clinics evolved away from a somewhat narrow preoccupation with the prevention of juvenile delinquency to a more general interest in the examination and treatment of parent–child relationships. Each clinic was staffed by a part-time psychiatrist, who served as director, a full-time psychologist, and three social workers. Each member of this "team" worked psychotherapeutically to some degree. While psychiatrists carried out any psychotherapy with the children that was deemed necessary, the psychologist often treated children with learning problems that the psychologist had diagnosed, and the social workers attempted to shape the attitudes of the children's parents and teachers. This division of labor was significant in so far as it assigned a therapeutic role to those professionals without medical training and established a precedent for both inpatient and outpatient "teamwork" following the war.

World War II

World War II set the stage for a massive expansion of the incipient field of psychotherapy. From the very beginning of the war, psychiatrists played a role in setting the policy for

the psychological screening of recruits, evaluating maladjust-
ment among soldiers, treating the mentally ill within the
armed services, and educating officers and enlisted men and
women about "preventative" mental health. Initially Harry
Stack Sullivan and Winfred Overholser, both of whom were
schooled in psychoanalysis and were practitioners of the new
psychiatry, acted as consultants to the director of selective
service after Congress passed the Conscription Act of 1940 in
response to heightened German aggression in the European
theater. Sullivan and Overholser argued successfully that
every recruit should receive not only a physical examination
but a psychiatric one as well. They used as the basis for their
exhortation the legacy of the government's insufficient attention to psychological problems during World War I. The federal government had spent over $1 billion caring for the psy-
chiatric casualties of that war, and yet, on the eve of World
War II, more than half of all Veterans Administration (VA)
hospital beds were still occupied by these men. Through psychiatric screening, Sullivan and Overholser maintained, the
costs of psychological disability could be significantly reduced.
While they were not able to persuade the military to imple-
ment psychiatric screening at the local draft board level, as
they had wished, the military agreed to institute it at every
induction center. Further, it was Sullivan, Overholser, and
other like-minded, psychoanalytically oriented psychiatrists
who developed the screening guidelines by which each recruit
was judged to be fit or not for military service (Berube, 1990,
pp. 12–14).

Sullivan and Overholser's influence at the beginning of
the war was taken up by William Menninger at the end of
1943 when he became director of the Neuropsychiatric Consultants Division in the Office of the Surgeon General, where
Menninger was on equal footing with the directors of medicine and surgery. Menninger, utilizing his psychoanalytic
orientation, emphasized talking therapy as the major way of
ameliorating psychological problems evinced by members of
the armed services. He vociferously maintained that prompt
treatment by psychiatrists, clinical psychologists, psychiatric
social workers, or psychiatric nurses in individual or group
therapy could enable men and women who had become

unable to serve to resume their previously held military positions.

On December 7, 1941, there were 35 psychiatrists in the regular Army Medical Corps. By the end of the war, there were 2,400 doctors practicing psychiatry in the army and 700 in the navy (Berube, 1990, p. 150). Also practicing were 1,710 psychologists, over half of whom engaged in psychotherapy in addition to their traditional roles as diagnosticians (Reisman, 1976, p. 298). And psychiatric social workers, many of whom had received little formal training, were assigned to practically every installation where a psychiatrist worked (Menninger, 1967, p. 505). This staff was dispersed through every induction center, most domestic and overseas general military hospitals and evacuation hospitals, 36 basic training camps, all large transports and hospital ships that carried psychiatric patients, many disciplinary barracks, redistribution and separation centers, and the ten specialized hospitals devoted entirely to neuropsychiatry, five of which were primarily for neurotic patients and three of which were for psychotic patients (Menninger, 1967, p. 529).

During the war, this staff participated in the development and execution of some 10 million standardized psychological tests, the performance of 500 training camp psychiatric consultations per month that lasted at least one-half hour, the discharge of approximately 380,000 men and women from the armed forces for psychological disability, and the treatment of 1 million patients in army hospitals (Menninger, 1967, pp. 503, 530; Reisman, 1976, p. 271). With the assistance of civilian psychiatrists, army psychiatrists examined approximately 15 million men at induction centers throughout the country before the war's end (Menninger, 1967, p. 531).

World War II thus had the effect of introducing literally millions of people to some form of psychological intervention for the first time in their lives. The war expanded the number of people involved in clinical practice through the army's training programs in psychiatry for physicians, through the army's active recruitment of psychiatrists, clinical psychologists, and psychiatric social workers directly out of medical and graduate schools, and through the army's training of military nurses and soldiers to be psychiatric nurses and psychiatric social workers.

While World War II clearly benefited the emerging field of psychotherapy more than any other event, it, however, did not result in immediate gains for women practitioners. Of the 2,400 doctors who served as psychiatrists during the war, only 16 were women. Of the 1,710 psychologists, only 40 were women; and out of those 40, only 20 were used to provide services to the military (Capshew & Laszlo, 1986, pp. 170–171). In fact, psychology was explicit in its rejection of women's direct participation in the war effort.

By the fall of 1940, psychologists had formed the Emergency Committee in Psychology (ECP) to bring to bear psychological expertise to aid the federal government in fighting the war. Its membership was exclusively male and heavily weighted with academic rather than clinical psychologists. It supported an Office of Psychological Personnel, however, to serve as an employment agency for psychologists seeking military and government positions. But because work in support of the war was considered a "man's job," women psychologists' potential contribution was denied. Despite many women's objection to this bias, they were informed that it was the woman's role to "keep the home fires burning" and to "wait, weep, and comfort one another" (quoted in Capshew & Laszlo, 1986, p. 163). The male leadership of the ECP told female psychologists to find *volunteer* work as a means of supporting the war effort, even though male psychologists were finding *paid* employment serving both the military and federal government.

In response to this discrimination, after Pearl Harbor women formed the National Council of Women Psychologists. Their purpose was a conciliatory one, explicitly not "militant-suffragist in tone," and not formed to protest their exclusion from mobilization committees and government positions. Rather they simply wanted a forum for women psychologists to promote specific projects in support of the war (Capshew & Laszlo, 1986, pp. 164–165). By the middle of 1942, the Council had 234 members, but because they focused their energies on civilian work, they accomplished little in gaining employment for female psychologists in the government or military. They performed some psychological testing for local selective service boards, evaluated and helped place volunteers in civilian defense agencies, and circulated course guides for the general populace on topics such as encouraging mothers to feed babies normally despite wartime conditions. But the Council did nothing to help women replace men in either academic or clinical employment settings, and it sat by idly as the unemployment rate of female psychologists actually increased during the war.

By 1947, the Council essentially disbanded. While leaving little of significance as its legacy, the existence of the National Council of Women Psychologists highlights the explicit discrimination against women in the field of psychology up through the end of World War II. It also reveals the small degree to which even the most disgruntled women were willing to pursue the fight against this discrimination. Thoroughly socialized into an elite scientific and professional perspective toward themselves and their world, they saw their low status as a reflection of idiosyncratic low achievement rather than discrimination based on gender (Capshew & Laszlo, 1986, p. 176).

Psychiatry and Psychology after the War

The war, however, did empower psychiatry as a profession. Never before had it experienced such influence and recognition from the federal government and from the public. Many psychiatrists saw the postwar period as an opportunity to continue to expand psychiatry's influence far beyond its traditional domain of the hospital and analytic consulting room. At the first meeting of the American Psychiatric Association after the war, William Menninger (1967), who had tasted real power as the army's chief psychiatric consultant, declared:

> To some of us psychiatry seems to be at a crossroads: we may continue to permit our chief emphasis of interest to be in the

psychoses or in seeing six or eight analytic patients a day in our ivory towers. . . . On the other hand, we can turn up the road that leads us into the broad field of social interests; we can devote our efforts to the potential opportunities of helping the average man on the street. We can reorganize our front on the basis that we have just experienced an international psychosis and we are living in a world filled with its residual of grief and sorrow and suffering that have nothing to do with "dementia praecox" or the "Oedipus conflict," but with individual struggles, community needs, state and national problems, and international concerns. (p. 538)

This call to engage in what was referred to as "social psychiatry" conceptually opened the door for the field of psychotherapy.[1] Rather than seeing potential patients only among the psychotic and the well-heeled neurotic who could afford psychoanalysis, Menninger spoke of the "average man on the street" whose problems were neither biologically determined nor products of deep unconscious conflict accessible only through free association. Because of the serious disruptions in everyone's lives due to the war, he believed there was a tremendous need psychiatry could fill in ameliorating the common person's suffering. Such amelioration could occur not only through direct clinical services but through public education and consultation to the criminal justice system, the public school system, and industry. He envisioned a preventative mental health movement that, if properly supported, could impact the public's mental health in a comparable fashion to how vaccination had transformed the spread of infectious disease (Menninger, 1967).

These goals remained beyond reach, however, if the demand for clinicians continued to far exceed supply. At the close of the war there were 37,000 "neuropsychiatric" casualties being treated in domestic government hospitals. Seven months later that number increased to 44,000 as more troops were demobilized and overseas hospitals dismantled. Due to

[1]Elmer Ernest Southard, one of the original "new psychiatrists" and Karl Menninger's mentor, originally coined the term "social psychiatry" in 1917, but it had dropped out of usage by 1925 (Levine, 1981, p. 34).

the huge number of draftees who were rejected for psychiatric reasons during the war (1,825,000, or 14% of all draftees), the large number who sought psychiatric assistance in basic training camp (between 4% to 5% of all men in basic training), and the number of psychiatric disabilities resulting from the war, the public became increasingly concerned about mental health and increasingly open to looking to psychiatric experts for help (Hilgard, 1987; Menninger, 1967). That help, however, was in short supply. Therefore the Veterans Administration made mental health services and training a cornerstone of its expanding operations. After the war, the VA began a construction program that ultimately led to the building of 69 general hospitals, each with a psychiatric unit, and 16 psychiatric hospitals (Friedman, 1990, p. 172). By 1955 the VA operated 41 psychiatric hospitals throughout the country (Albee, 1959, p. 36). More importantly, the VA instituted a large training program for both psychiatrists and clinical psychologists. And it extended the psychologist's official duties to include psychotherapy, thus expanding clinical psychology beyond its traditional domain of expertise in testing and diagnosis.

At the request of the VA and the U.S. Public Health Service, which sought to meet the mental health needs of the large number of returning veterans, the American Psychological Association (APA) developed a model for clinical psychology training programs. Called the "scientist–practitioner" model, it was devised at a conference in Boulder, Colorado, convened by the American Psychological Association in August 1949. This form of training continues today as the model for the education of most doctoral level clinical psychologists. For the first time the APA acknowledged psychotherapy as an officially sanctioned component of a clinical psychologist's function that requires serious academic instruction. But the APA insisted that prior to practicing as a psychotherapist, a clinical psychologist had to master a course of study in the "science" of psychology and demonstrate sufficient research capabilities before being granted a doctoral degree. Thus, under pressure from the federal government to formulate standards for the training of psychotherapists, the APA officially granted a place for psychotherapy within academia. But because of its firm entrenchment and roots within positivist science and the university, the APA made sure that practitioners formed an allegiance to academic psychology.

Psychiatry's wariness of clinical psychologists' ability to treat patients in the absence of medical training, coupled with the APA's attempt to control the education of psychotherapists placed the newly formed field of clinical psychology in an awkward professional position. Fox, Kovacs, and Graham (1985) describe the field as the "illegitimate child of psychiatry and academic psychology—parents who have always viewed its development with fear, suspicion, and ambivalence" (p. 1043). Due to these attitudes, clinical psychology has attempted since 1949 to carve out a professional niche for itself somewhere between psychotherapy practice, which originated in psychiatry, and academic psychology, which continues to dictate its educational requirements.

In addition to the official recognition of clinical psychology, the increased interest in mental health due to the war prompted Congress in 1946 to pass a National Mental Health Act, thereby creating an agency to be called the National Institute of Mental Health (NIMH). NIMH, which came to fruition in 1949, was to promote mental health as well as oversee the care of the mentally ill. To this end it provided training grants to students of psychiatry, clinical psychology, psychiatric social work, and psychiatric nursing.

Therefore, within only a few years following the end of the war, a solid foundation for the training of professionals who were to provide direct clinical services was firmly in place. The VA provided training facilities and faculty, funding for trainees, and job opportunities for graduates of its clinical programs; and the NIMH allocated research grants and fellowships to students within universities.

Psychodynamics: The American Invention

The backbone of what these increasing numbers of trainees and residents learned in their training programs at the VA and elsewhere was one form or another of psychoanalytic theory and technique. Partly due to the influence of Sullivan, Over-holser, Menninger, and others during the war, a psychoanalytic understanding—however diluted—appeared to be the salient paradigm of thought both during and immediately following the war. Thousands of former military doctors pressured the VA to provide them with psychiatric training after the war. These physicians as well as clinical psychology trainees and psychiatric residents were sent to training facilities that were predominantly psychoanalytic in orientation, such as the Menninger School of Psychiatry, which trained half the psychiatrists in the VA system and one third of all psychiatric residents in the United States in the postwar period (Friedman, 1990, pp. 174, 176). Due to the success of William Menninger in shaping the army's psychiatric policies during the war and the sway psychoanalytic training programs held in the VA, psychoanalytic psychotherapy appeared to be the wave of the future to those in the federal training system.

Psychoanalytic thinking was enhanced further by the influx of psychoanalysts into the United States due to the rise of the Third Reich and the ensuing dislocations as Hitler's troops marched across Europe in the 1930s and 1940s. By the end of the war, the center of psychoanalytic thought had shifted from Europe to the United States. Psychoanalytic émigrés brought a new vitality to training programs, psychoanalytic institutes, and professional journals and conferences, as they spread across the country from their typical point of immigration in New York (Hale, 1978).

Partially as a consequence of the rising popularity of the psychoanalytic framework, many analysts began moving away from strict analytic technique toward the practice of analytically informed psychotherapy, or "psychodynamic psychotherapy," as it became known after the war. Due to the widespread interest in treating greater numbers of patients from different social classes and different diagnostic categories, many psychoanalytically oriented practitioners saw patients less frequently than the typical four or five times a week mandated by psychoanalysis and treated them more supportively, with less of an emphasis on interpretation (Alexander & French, 1946; Fromm-Reichmann, 1950; Gill, 1954, 1984).

By 1952, the widespread acceptance of a psychoanalytic framework was reflected in a very influential NIMH-supported American Psychiatric Association Conference on Psychiatric Education held at Cornell University. In its book of proceedings, the Conference concluded that: "It is now almost universally agreed that a necessary part of the preparation of a competent psychiatrist is the development of and understanding of principles of psychodynamics," and that "it seems obvious that an understanding of psychodynamics presupposes—indeed necessitates— . . . knowledge of Freudian concepts and of psychoanalytic theory and practice" (quoted in Wallerstein, 1989, p. 566).

Robert Wallerstein (1989) points out that psychoanalytically informed psychotherapy, in its widespread application following World War II, was a distinctively American innovation.[2] While psychoanalysis proper was practiced in both Europe and Latin America at the time, nowhere else was Freudian *psychotherapy* a focus of practice or a theorized field. Certainly nowhere else in the world did it form the foundation of both psychiatric residencies and clinical psychologists' internships and postdoctoral training programs.

The popularity and acceptance of a psychoanalytic understanding fell upon the fertile ground of postwar prosperity. Freed from the economic exigencies of the depression and World War II, more Americans than ever before could turn their attentions to personal problems, doubts, and desires that

---

[2]Wallerstein (1989) points out that psychodynamic psychotherapy is, in fact, the only uniquely American contribution to the field of psychiatry.

> Psychoanalysis was created by Freud in Austria; the descriptive nosology of the major mental disorders was the work of Kraepelin and his school in Germany; electroconvulsive therapy was inaugurated by Cerletti and Bini in Italy, insulin coma by Sakel in Hungary, and the ill-starred lobotomy operation by Egas Moniz in Portugal; the concept of the therapeutic community was developed by Maxwell Jones in England; the modern psychoactive drug era was inaugurated in Switzerland with Largactil, later brought to America as Thorazine; and lithium was first successfully employed by Cade in Australia. (p. 566)

had been shadowed in the 1930s by a national economy in ruins and in the 1940s by a total social mobilization to support the war. By the end of the 1950s, psychoanalytic explanation and jargon pervaded middle-class culture in the United States, and psychotherapy, the uniquely American phenomenon, was a growing, prosperous field. John Seeley could announce in his famous article of 1961, "The Americanization of the Unconscious," that there had occurred a

> "psychoanalyzation" of American thought, institutions, and life. . . . This development in America, and it has still to run the major part of its course, makes for a change in the very nature of the society, comparable to the original American Revolution. But that was a revolution of mere *externa*: this is of *interna, ultima, privatissima*. (pp. 191, 198)

While the psychoanalytic paradigm was dominant in the postwar period in terms of the development of psychotherapy as a field, it was not hegemonic. It was challenged from two quite different quarters. First, Carl Rogers had offered an original form of counseling or psychotherapy immediately before the war in his book *The Clinical Treatment of the Problem Child* (1939). He developed his ideas more thoroughly and applied them to the treatment of adults in his highly influential *Counseling and Psychotherapy* (1942). His "client-centered therapy" rested on a theory and technique developed exclusively for psychotherapy. This stood in contradistinction to psychoanalysis, which always viewed psychotherapy as its poor relation, unworthy of a customized theory or technique that was anything more than watered-down analysis. Rogerian therapy became immensely popular. Rogers was elected president of the APA in 1947. His views were particularly salient in a number of university-based psychology departments and in counseling psychology and clinical social work training programs. His was the first widely accepted theory of psychotherapy that originated outside psychoanalysis and that conceptualized psychotherapy as a field in its own right. He paved the way for the burgeoning of psychotherapeutic theories and techniques that successfully challenged the dominance of psychoanalysis in the 1960s.

Second, the discovery of Thorazine in 1950 and its marketing in the United States beginning in 1954 ushered in a new age of biological psychiatry, which had been declining in influence for many years. Within two years after its introduction to the American market, doctors were prescribing Thorazine to 2 million patients, and psychoactive drugs were widely seen as the panacea for severe mental disturbance. In 1955 Congress unanimously passed a resolution, the Mental Health Study Act, to provide for "an objective, thorough, and nationwide analysis and reevaluation of the human and economic problems of mental illness" (quoted in Levine, 1981, p. 46). Six years later the committee that carried out this analysis, the Joint Commission on Mental Illness and Health, concluded that psychoactive drugs "have revolutionized the management of psychotic patients in American mental hospitals, and probably deserve primary credit for reversal of the upward spiral of the State hospital inpatient load" (quoted in Scull, 1977, p. 81). Therefore, within only 7 years, drug therapy had become the treatment of choice for psychosis in vast numbers of mental hospitals throughout the United States. While private hospitals with firm roots in psychoanalytic tradition used psychotropic drugs sparingly and typically only in conjunction with psychotherapy, increasing numbers of state hospitals used them exclusively. They were inexpensive and exerted a tranquilizing effect on psychotic symptoms, thus making the management of what were often unruly patients much easier for staff. The introduction of the phenothiazines in the 1950s thus presaged what would emerge as the greatest challenge to the field of psychotherapy in the ensuing decades, namely one form or another of drug therapy.

The New Frontier of Mental Health Care

As in so many aspects of our social and professional lives, the 1960s heralded change in mental health care practice that exceeded in its swiftness, intensity, and magnitude anything previously witnessed in the history of psychotherapy. In 1960 the state mental hospital remained the chief feature of mental health care delivery in the United States, despite steady decreases in the hospital census since 1955. In 1961 the Joint Commission on Mental Illness and Health recommended that these hospitals be phased out and that a nationwide system of community mental health centers be erected in their place. It was this report that prompted President Kennedy to address Congress in February 1963, calling for a

> wholly new emphasis and approach to care for the mentally ill. This approach relies primarily upon the new knowledge and new drugs acquired and developed in recent years which make it possible for most of the mentally ill to be successfully and quickly treated in their own communities and returned to a useful place in society. . . .
>
> I am convinced that, if we apply our medical knowledge and social insights fully, all but a small portion of the mentally ill can eventually achieve a wholesome and constructive social adjustment. (quoted in Buckhout, 1971, p. 375)

Based in an extremely optimistic and exuberent sense of possibility, Kennedy proposed to Congress "a broad new mental health program" built around "the essential concept of the comprehensive community mental health center" that would

> focus community resources and provide better community facilities for all aspects of mental health care. Prevention as well as treatment will be a major activity. Located in the patient's own environment and community, the center would make possible a better understanding of his needs, a more cordial atmosphere for his recovery and a continuum of treatment. . . .
>
> When carried out, reliance on the cold mercy of custodial isolation will be supplanted by the open warmth of community concern and capability. Emphasis on prevention, treatment and rehabilitation will be substituted for a desultory interest in confining patients in an institution to wither away. (quoted in Buckhout, 1971, p. 375)

Kennedy's exhortation resulted in the 1963 passage by Congress of the Community Mental Health Centers Construction Act. This act committed the federal government to a policy of shifting support away from the large state mental institutions to community-based centers, which employed all professional categories of mental health practitioners and which placed psychotherapy, along with drug therapy, at the foundation of the services provided. These centers were not intended to serve only the psychotic, as the state mental hospital had done, or primarily men, as the VA hospitals did, or largely the middle and upper-middle classes, the traditional recipients of psychoanalysis. By law these centers were mandated to treat anyone within their community regardless of diagnosis, prognosis, age, sex, race, or ability to pay. In many ways they represented an outgrowth of the social psychiatry movement in that their goals were both clinical and, to a lesser degree, preventative and educational.

In order to receive federal funding, the community mental health centers were required to provide a mix of services: inpatient facilities for short-term hospitalizations; outpatient psychotherapy for adults and children; 24-hour crisis intervention; outreach programs to attract those who might otherwise not know about or be amenable to mental health servies; day treatment programs so those with severe mental disorders could reside within their communities rather than in state mental hospitals; drug and alcohol rehabilitation; consultation services for schools, businesses, and institutions in an effort to provide education about preventative mental health care; and research and program evaluation to determine centers' effectiveness.

Although its funding was always inadequate, the community mental health system had the effect of introducing large numbers of people to psychotherapy. Between 1957 and 1976, the percentage of the population using professional mental health services increased from 14% to 26% (Kiesler & Morton, 1988, p. 998). Outpatient mental health services increased twelvefold (Kiesler, 1982, p. 1323). By 1975 there were over 500 federally funded community mental health centers operating in the United States (Levine, 1981, p. 63). Far more than the mental hospital or the Upper East Side analytic consulting room, the workplace for psychotherapy during these years was located in the community mental health clinic.

As the state mental hospitals were emptied of patients who were directed to community mental health centers, and as the acceptance of psychotherapy grew among increasing segments of the population, the demand for trained clinicians far outpaced supply. Since the end of the war, clinical psychology had become increasingly identified with the practice of psychotherapy. Now, as the demand for psychotherapists grew, psychiatric social workers took on the role of psychotherapists within mental health clinics. Between 1947 and 1977 there was a fivefold increase among mental health professionals. The number of psychiatrists and licensed clinical psychologists per 100,000 people in the population increased by a factor of ten within 30 years (Kiesler & Morton, 1988). Yet by the mid-1970s the demand for psychotherapists remained high, and training programs, at all professional levels, did not yet satisfy this need.

Throughout the 1970s health care costs in general began to rise, as did the cost of outpatient mental health care services. In 1967 outpatient or "ambulatory" services, which includes psychotherapy, accounted for less than 1% of all reimbursements for health care. By the close of the 1970s this had increased to 12%. Still, outpatient services only accounted for $30 million in reimbursements, while inpatient psychiatric services, despite deinstitutionalization, accounted for close to $100 million (Klerman, 1983, p. 932). Nevertheless, interest in cost containment for mental health outpatient services and growing questions about the efficacy of psychotherapy became a policy interest of the Carter administration. Fueled by the tremendous expansion of mental health utilization and of the number of mental health practitioners, in 1977 President Carter created the President's Commission on Mental Health to review the federal programs related to mental health, with particular emphasis on the future of the community mental health movement. Based on the report of this commission, in 1978 the Mental Health Systems Act was formulated and passed by Congress. It called for increased emphasis on community-based networks of care and new resources for both treatment and research. It renewed the federal government's commitment to comprehensive care and stressed the importance of targeting underserved geographical areas, serving low-income people, and gaining the participation of local citizens to serve on the boards of community mental health clinics.

"Endangered" Psychotherapy

Federal commitment to the community mental health system, however, shifted radically with the election of Ronald Reagan in 1980. In fact, the federal government's commitment to funding any form of mental health care began a sharp spiral downward at this time. Reagan's presidency, along with a number of other developments, challenged the field of psychotherapy on a variety of fronts. After three decades of growth, the 1980s stands as a decade of reversal, compromise, and significantly lowered expectations for psychotherapists and their clients.

Before the Mental Health Systems Act could even take effect, it was repealed, and the Omnibus Reconciliation Act of 1981 was passed. The Reconciliation Act cut federal funds for mental health services by 25%. In place of the Systems Act, the Reagan administration moved the Alcohol, Drug Abuse and Mental Health Block Grant through Congress in 1981, signaling abdication of the federal government's responsibility for the mentally ill. Under this legislation, individual states have discretion in determining to what use their block grants will be put, and the states are under no obligation to report in detail about their mental health services or policies to the federal government. Thus, due to budget needs or ideological preferences, states can determine that their federal block grant monies be removed from child crisis psychotherapy services to cocaine dependency programs, or vice versa, without violating any federal mandates.

Due to increasing health care costs in general and the growing number of Americans who do not have any form of health insurance or who are underinsured, the 1980s witnessed a dramatic rise in calls for some form of national health care coverage. Yet in all the reform bills submitted to Congress, mental health care has fallen to the bottom of the priority list. What is typically specified in a variety of bills is 45 days of inpatient care and 20 outpatient visits per calendar year. However, in a widely circulated Paine Webber report that has had a significant effect on the way Congress is thinking about national health coverage, "Nationalized Health Care in the 1990s," the company predicts that the federal government will adopt some form of national health insurance during the 1990s and mental health coverage probably will not be included (Wagner, 1991, pp. 1, 27).

The federal government's abdication for overseeing mental health care delivery has placed the onus of responsibility for outpatient treatment on states, third-party payers (insurance companies), and clients themselves. Due to the increasing magnitude of fiscal crisis in states, and particularly in those states that have witnessed some of the highest utilization rates for psychotherapy (e.g., New York, Massachusetts, California), cutbacks have affected virtually all community mental health centers. Many have closed entirely, cut back services and personnel, reduced hours, merged with other units, limited the number of psychotherapy visits, and/or limited the kinds of clients seen. As staff has been scaled back, drugs have increasingly been relied upon as a means of controlling symptoms rather than facilitating the process of psychotherapy. The monitoring of medications takes 15 minutes once every month or two. Psychotherapy requires at least a 45- or 50-minute hour once a week over a period of weeks, months, or years.

With the decline in federal and state support for outpatient mental health services, practitioners in the dwindling public sector have come to rely increasingly on hospitalization. Insurance companies typically pay for hospitalizations but not for outpatient treatment or nonmedical forms of residential care. This applies to the federal government's Medicaid program as well, insofar as almost 80% of its Medicaid funds are spent on state mental hospitalizations, leaving little for community-based services (Dougherty, 1988, pp. 809–810).

In the private sector, in an attempt to contain reimbursement costs, insurers have significantly scaled back psychotherapy benefits while continuing to cover psychiatric hospitalization. Most recently insurers have acted to curtail the length of hospitalizations as well. Increasingly insurance companies are permitting hospital stays of no more than 2 weeks, thus bringing the average stay in a private psychiatric hospital down to around 20 days ("The Squeeze on Psychiatric Chains," 1991).

While third-party payers continue to view psychiatric hospitalizations as a necessary medical expense that must be contained and meted out sparingly, psychotherapy is now seen simply as a luxury in an era when expenditures for mental health care have been rising twice as fast as general medical costs (Zimet, 1989, p. 704). Yet in reality psychotherapy remains a small part of the spiraling figures often quoted in the media. Despite the fact that outpatient psychotherapy consistently represents only 3% to 4% of the nation's annual health care expenditures, insurance carriers continue to maintain that coverage for psychotherapy increases people's utilization of services and contributes to the fact that health care costs now stand at 11% of the gross national product, whereas in 1960 they represented only 5%.

As important as this misguided belief regarding utilization is the carriers' inability to evaluate psychotherapy services. Because they do not fall easily into a medical model, such services stymie insurers simply because "cure" is so difficult to determine. While it is well established that typical medical treatments, such as appendectomies, allergy shots, or radiation therapy for breast cancer involve an average number of interventions over a specified amount of time, psychotherapy can seem indeterminate. Because there is no clear disease process being treated and no absolute standard of treatment, carriers increasingly view psychotherapy as a financial vortex to avoid in an era of escalating health care expenditures.

According to Carl Zimet (1989), without direct linkage between diagnosis and type of treatment, schedule of treatment, or length of treatment, and being unable to clearly fit into the bounds of

> medical necessity . . . , outpatient psychotherapy falls into the endangered reimbursement category. . . .
> It is unhappily altogether conceivable that coverage for outpatient psychotherapy could be eliminated from insurance plans just as cosmetic surgery has been excluded, and full payment would come directly from the patients. . . . A return to the era before health insurance provided coverage of outpatient treatment would mean that psychotherapy would be available only to the affluent. (p. 706)

This pessimistic scenario is mirrored in managed health care, which is best represented by the preferred provider organization (PPO) and the health maintenance organization (HMO). Managed care is increasingly caring for Americans' health care needs. In 1980, 9.1 million people were enrolled in HMOs; by 1992, 35 to 39 million were, and as many as 65 million people were cared for by PPOs (Wylie, 1992c, p. 34). In order to be licensed as federally qualified, an HMO must at least provide short-term psychotherapy. "Short-term" is defined as not exceeding 20 visits. Because HMOs are structured to limit the procedures that are not of medical necessity (given their prepaid, fixed payment basis), many HMOs actually provide their enrollees with far less than the 20 visits mandated by federal statute. This, in fact, is the practice of the 12 HMOs I surveyed in Northern California. While two of the HMOs have "extended" plans available that offer 50 sessions with relatively generous criteria for being seen in psychotherapy, their regular health coverage, along with the plans of the 10 others surveyed, state that a client can be seen for 20 sessions. In practice, however, a person must be suffering a major situational crisis to be seen for any more than 6 sessions. That this information is not available to enrollees of these HMOs and is left to the individual psychotherapist to announce during a client's first psychotherapy session is apparently uniform practice among the dozen organizations surveyed.

Rather than being anomalous, such practice is logical in the HMO prepaid health delivery system. This system seeks to enlarge its membership base *and* control costs through minimizing its members' utilization of the system, and particularly their use of medical specialists (e.g., anyone apart from the primary care physician who acts as the HMO gatekeeper). Rogers Wright, director of the Association for the Advancement of Psychology and an expert on mental health reimbursement issues, frames the issue concisely:

> Managed care relies on disincentives to care. Participants in the program are rewarded for not providing care. When you as a provider go into a system in which your rewards are based on *not* delivering care, you better believe you're not going to deliver as much care as an independent provider. (quoted in Wylie, 1992c, p. 37)

Within HMOs, just as in hospitals, clinics, and private consulting rooms, psychiatrists are also increasingly turning away from the practice of psychotherapy for reasons both related to and independent of the issues raised by managed care. Since the development of Thorazine in the early 1950s, a steady stream of new psychoactive drugs has been invented to ameliorate the symptoms of ever-greater numbers of psychological disorders. Initially psychosis was the major target of drug therapy, but with the development of both Lithium and antidepressants, mood disorders of both acute and chronic duration have been increasingly treated with medications. Now personality disorders, phobias, eating disorders, panic attacks, and compulsive disorders, such as kleptomania, are in many cases being treated by antidepressants as well. The cover story from the July 6, 1992 issue of *Time* magazine, "Pills for the Mind," reflects this enthusiasm. "It is the psychopharmacologists," the article boldly asserts, "who are making the breakthroughs in mental-health circles," and *not* the psychotherapists (Elmer-Dewitt, 1992, p. 58).

Researchers increasingly are finding genetically based

abnormalities to account for various forms of mental illness. Molecular biologists are beginning to map abnormal behavior to specific strands of DNA. And by following the action of drugs like Clozapine for schizophrenia and Prozac for depression, moods can be linked to the actions of particular neurotransmitters (Elmer-Dewitt, 1992, p. 58). The findings of this research are not merely disseminated in professional journals but are frequently reported in the media for mass consumption. A recent article from the *Los Angeles Times*, and picked up by many other newspapers throughout the country, cites a "landmark study" sponsored by the National Institute of Child Health and Human Development:

> The long-awaited study, the most definitive in a long series trying to separate the effects of genetics and environment in a child's development, comes down heavily on the side of genetics.
> It indicates that the broad outlines of personality and behavior are put in place in the brief instant of conception, establishing the basic route that the child will take during the rest of its life. . . .
> "For most every behavioral trait so far investigated, from reaction time to religiosity, an important fraction of the variation among people turns out to be associated with genetic variation," wrote the University of Minnesota researchers. ("NIMH Landmark Study," 1990).

The belief in a biologic basis to behavior and psychopathology infuses the practice of psychiatry and, increasingly, the public's perception of mental illness. The inherent form of treatment that follows from this understanding is pharmacologic, rather than psychotherapeutic. This viewpoint flourishes in an age of dwindling resources for helping the mentally ill. Drug therapy, because it takes so little time to prescribe and monitor, is considerably cheaper than psychotherapy, so that the state, third-party payers and managed forms of health care increasingly endorse drug therapy as the treatment of choice. Since the public is routinely exposed to biologic explanations of mental illness, and since the lure of a quick fix or magic pill is unquestionably appealing, few clients or their families are motivated to question this approach.

Psychiatry benefits from this trend. It alone among mental health professions has drug prescribing privileges. As the number of clinical psychologists and social workers continues to increase, and all three professional groupings compete more or less equally in the outpatient psychotherapy market, psychiatrists can remain distinct, their professional identity intact, through prescribing medications. Therefore, in line with the current research, funding patterns, and psychiatry's desire to maintain its competitive edge, psychiatric residencies throughout the country are abandoning training in psychotherapy in favor of an emphasis on psychopharmacology and neurophysiology.

Thus in the last decade of the 20th century, the field of psychotherapy is being strenuously challenged, in marked contrast with its much more secure status only 15 years ago. Due to cutbacks in both state funding and third-party payments, the rise of managed health care, the decline of the community mental health system, and a growing emphasis on psychopharmacology, psychotherapy has become "endangered," as Carl Zimet declares (1989, p. 706). The occupation now being feminized bears little resemblance to the robust and expanding field that grew to maturity in the 1960s and 1970s. And it is in this transformation that feminization, as we shall see, is anchored.

A Perfect Match?:
Women and Psychotherapy

The field of psychotherapy has increasingly become endangered, just as the pool of potential women workers available to fill and expand its ranks has sharply increased. This interesting coincidence of historical trajectories—psychotherapy's decreasing status and women's greater availability to enter the field—underlies the process of feminization at its core.

In order to understand the complex relationship between these two historical processes, we first need to look at women's labor force participation in general. Simply stated, throughout the 20th century, women's labor force participation has risen. During the last three decades that rise has been dramatic. In 1960, 37.8% of all the nation's working-age women were in the labor force; by 1990, the number had risen to 57.7%. This contrasts with a gradual decline in men's participation rates. In 1960, 84% of all working-age men were in the labor force; by 1990, this had dropped to 75.6%.

Women's increased participation has been fueled by a number of historically unprecedented factors. First, demographic shifts have made possible increased participation rates. In general, women are having fewer children and therefore fewer child rearing responsibilities, permitting them longer time in the paid labor force. This trend, however, is not simply unilateral because women's greater labor force participation appears to further reduce women's expected fertility and its concomitant level of family responsibilities. Thus, decreased birth rates allow greater labor force participation, and, in turn, increased participation rates tend to exert a negative effect on birth rates.

Second, for married couples and two-parent families to maintain a relatively constant standard of living over time, it has become necessary for wives and mothers to work outside the home. During the 1980s, real wages fell after adjusting for inflation. Between 1978 and 1988, the average hourly wage fell from $11.27 an hour to $10.13 (measured in constant 1990 dollars). For young men in the 25- to 34-year-old age group—when men have typically married and begun families—median income fell from $26,879 in 1973 to $20,782 in 1988 (measured in 1988 dollars). In order to maintain a family's standard of living, increasing numbers of married women have entered the paid labor force. This trend is reflected in the fact that the women exhibiting the greatest increase in labor force participation in recent years have been those who have been traditionally least likely to work outside the home—married women with young children (Roos, 1985, p. 14).

Another indication of this trend is mirrored in the fact that the proportion of salaried families with only one worker fell by more than one half between 1950 and 1980 (Brown, 1987, p. 20). Currie, Dunn, and Fogarty (1990) term this trend "social speedup resembling the deliberately increased pace of an industrial assembly line" (p. 323). Just to maintain a standard of living over time, more family members are forced out into the paid labor force. This in turn

> often means a decline in the possibility of real leisure—or, what amounts to the same thing, an increase in the pace of life. . . .
> Most of the extra work brought by the speedup has fallen on women, because they are most of the second earners in the paid labor force and because paid work has not freed most women from unpaid work at home. (p. 323)

According to Clair Brown (1987), beginning in the 1970s, whether or not a wife works outside the home became a chief means of distinguishing families' ability to withstand economic downturns. Within each social class she examined, a significant income differential existed between those families that had a wife employed in the labor force and those that did not (Brown, 1987, p. 31). Thus a wife's ability to work outside the home became a critical variable in determining a family's income and its chances for both weathering recessions and inflation and moving up or down within its social class.

Social speedup or the need for two-earner families is fundamentally intertwined with a third factor relating to women's increased participation rates, namely, the demise of the family wage. By the early 20th century, the American economy was premised on the family wage. Male workers had fought for and won the right to be paid enough to support a family. The family wage rested on the assumption of a division of labor in which men worked outside the home for money, and women worked within the home performing unremunerated domestic labor and child rearing. Implicit in the idea of the family wage were the assumptions that men freely chose to support women and children with it and that women were paid considerably less than men if they entered the paid labor force because they did not have to support families. Although single, divorced, deserted, and widowed women typically suffered under this regime, the family wage system worked for many if not most families during the greater part of the 20th century. "In fact," notes author Barbara Ehrenreich (1983), "considering the absence of legal coercion, the surprising thing is that men have for so long, and, on the whole, so reliably, adhered to what we might call the 'breadwinner ethic'" (p. 11).

In the past 20 years, the breadwinner ethic has experienced a radical reversal. As will be shown at length in Chapter 6, men are increasingly unwilling to freely support women and children. Through postponement of marriage, a preference for women who will not become financially dependent, divorce, and an alarming widespread refusal to pay spousal and child support, men have "revolted," to use Ehrenreich's (1983) term, against the breadwinner ethic.

In the space of a few decades, our culture has inverted the expectations that made the family wage system in any sense justifiable as a means of distributing wealth from those who are relatively advantaged as wage earners to many of those (women and children) who are not. Men still have the incentives to work and even to succeed at dreary and manifestly useless jobs, but not necessarily to work *for others*. (p. 12)

Seen from this perspective, the family wage system has broken down not only because one income no longer permits families to retain a consistent standard of living but also due to men's increasing reluctance to share the relatively greater incomes they do earn with women and children. Therefore the legacy of the family wage is the fact that men continue to make more money than women in the paid labor force (as discussed in Chapter 1), but the corresponding moral and cultural assumption that they freely support economic dependents has more or less evaporated.

Short of a program to conscript men into marriage and (in recalcitrant cases) have male earnings deposited directly to their wives' accounts, women have no sure claim on the wages of men. For women as a group, the future holds terrifying insecurity: We are increasingly dependent on our own resources, but in a society and an economy that never intended to admit us as independent persons, much less as breadwinners for others. (Ehrenreich, 1983, p. 175)

The collapse of the family wage system by necessity has forced increasing numbers of women into the paid labor force. Because of this collapse, few women today can expect to be adequately supported by a man for any significant portion of their lives. While in previous historic times this expectation might have been viewed only in terms of economic hardship (and for many women still is), the contemporary feminist movement has provided women with a means of understanding participation in the paid labor force as an avenue toward self-realization and fulfillment, independence from men, and potential liberation from constricting and dehumanizing sex roles.

"Second-wave" feminists have consistently critiqued women's absolute identification with the domestic sphere and heralded employment outside the home as a means to equality with men. Refusing to accept the kinds of work women did outside the home in the 1950s and early 1960s as the only possible outlets for women's paid employment, feminists in the late 1960s began arguing the case that there was virtually no job for which women were not suited or capable of performing. Feminists encouraged every woman to aspire to any job—from manual labor to the skilled trades to the highest echelons of professional work. And largely because of feminism's impact, they have.

As women graduate college, or contemplate returning to the labor force after an absence, or decide to change occupations after already establishing a career, working in any one of the professions has increasingly become an option women consider. For compelling reasons, the field of psychotherapy has become quite alluring for women who are considering a professional career.

Psychotherapy as the Professionalization of Motherhood

Psychotherapy's attractiveness to women is multifaceted. The working conditions, the form, and the content of the occupation all appear to be compatible with women's dual roles of labor force participant, on the one hand, and domestic worker and mother on the other.

The majority of psychotherapy practitioners today engage in private practice on either a full-time or part-time basis. Private practice, and even some salaried employment in clinic and hospital settings, permit therapists to set their own schedules. Such flexibility can amount to an absolute necessity for women who are trying to juggle child care and/or domestic chores with professional commitments. There is little other professional work that is so easily practiced in the evenings and weekends or for small and large blocks of time throughout the day depending on a practitioner's idiosyncratic needs.

Through private practice, a woman can work close to home or even in her own home. Since little more than two or three chairs are needed to set up a consulting room, office space can be readily found, and often for minimal rent. Increasingly therapists' offices are found outside of medical buildings in generic office buildings, houses, or apartment buildings that have been converted into therapy offices. The possibility of establishing a consulting room in any one of these venues is vast and therefore increases the likelihood that a woman can find office space close to home if that is her choice. Many practitioners also transform an extra bedroom, part of a living room, or an unused garage into an office in which to see clients. This makes possible a virtually effortless transition between women's dual roles.

Both private practice and salaried employment offer a certain amount of flexibility in case of a domestic emergency, such as a child's illness. Clients' appointments typically can be cancelled or rescheduled without irreparable damage, for in psychotherapy there are no deadlines to meet, no illnesses that require immediate solutions. Such flexibility also permits interruption due to therapists' pregnancies (albeit with complex consequences for clients). As the feminization of the field progresses, the professional literature on how to practically and psychologically handle pregnancy and maternity leaves within the framework of a psychotherapy treatment has vastly expanded.

But perhaps more important than these logistical attractions are the way the form and content of psychotherapeutic practice fits with what have been women's more traditional roles within the home. The form psychotherapy typically takes is that of two (and sometimes more) people sitting across from each other and talking in a homelike setting. As any tour of women's (and certainly some men's) psychotherapy offices reveals, consulting rooms often cannot easily be distinguished from parlors, studies, or living rooms. Comfortable chairs or couches, paintings on the walls, vases of flowers, and even fireplaces give the impression of domestic comfort. And within these cozy settings, therapists often sit in one chair for hours, patiently listening to and commenting upon others' problems, misfortunes, and the mundane vicissitudes of everyday life. Therefore, the outward form or appearance psychotherapy takes resembles what women—

particularly of the middle and upper classes—have done for centuries.

In her interviews with early women psychoanalysts, Nancy Chodorow (1991) found that "psychoanalytic practice felt, as some put it, 'natural for women' or a 'mothering profession,' as it required passive sitting, intuition and empathic understanding" (p. 14). The content of the work itself—talk or play therapy, empathic immersion in another's experience, containment of another's feelings and fantasies, the nonjudgmental acceptance of positive and negative transferences, provision of a "holding environment," maintenance of boundaries—bears a striking similarity to what women have always done, namely, rear children.[1] And this "motherly" work is often conceptualized in theories that focus on life within the family, that is, a realm of social experience for which women always have had a particular interest and expertise. Whether one practices from a psychodynamic, family systems, or "12-step" perspective (to name only a few), family life is theoretically privileged as the means of understanding human motivation and psychopathology.

It is also relevant to point out that the manner in which many women decide to become psychotherapists is through their own experience in psychotherapy with another woman, which is not entirely unlike the way daughters develop the capacities for mothering in their families of origin. Through their own experience of empathic immersion and continuity with their mothers, daughters develop both an ability and desire to become mothers themselves. It is in order to once again experience primary identification and a sense of self that is continuous with another that propels women to take responsibility for mothering from one generation to the next (Chodorow, 1978). Because women represent the majority of psychotherapy clients (Taube, Burns, & Kessler, 1984, p. 1438) and, increasingly, psychotherapy practitioners, the opportunities for women to work with female therapists have grown. And since the therapeutic relationship involves a

[1]Of course the way people now think about child rearing is itself influenced by a child rearing literature that historically has drawn upon psychodynamic theories.

similiar empathic immersion to that between mother and child, at its best, therapy can enable a woman client to feel fully recognized, understood, and helped. After experiencing a psychotherapy that has both elicited a rich transference relationship and promoted psychological growth, many women desire to recapitulate the relationship by becoming therapists themselves in a fashion similar to the way that daughters eventually choose to become mothers. As women contemplate career choices or changes, their intimate and often powerful experiences in their own psychotherapies provide them with very real, very close-at-hand knowledge of not only what psychotherapists *do* but how they *are*. In this sense, then, clients' identification with their therapists is "personal" rather than "positional." They identify with the actual personal attributes of their therapist rather than simply with the role or position she occupies in an occupational structure.

In the way that a daughter can identify not only with the various acts her mother performs in both child rearing and domestic work but her idiosyncratic attitudes and values toward and feelings about those acts, so too can a psychotherapy client identify with the real person of the therapist rather than a mere role about which she fantasizes.[2] While such personal identification can also take place in cross-gendered therapies—as when a woman sees a male therapist—it seems that the capacity to envision oneself as being *like* or *the same as* one's therapist *may* be greater in same-sex therapy arrangements. And certainly as women increasingly come to numerically dominate the field, it becomes more likely that a female client will see a female therapist. It makes sense, then, that as feminization continues, the occupational reproduction of women psychotherapists will proliferate.

Given how much psychotherapy seems to be a "motherly profession," what seems remarkable is not that women are coming to prevail within its ranks but rather that men

[2]It is not unusual for therapists to find themselves unself-consciously appropriating gestures, words, inflections, styles of speech, and various mannerisms of their current or past therapists into their own practice. Of course, it would be interesting to know empirically whether or not this occurs more frequently between same-sex client–therapist pairs.

have numerically dominated the profession for so long. It appears that as soon as women began to seek professional work outside the home in large numbers, a pool of potential female psychotherapists appeared. It only took the field of psychotherapy to welcome women into its ranks for the process of feminization to begin. And that seems to be exactly what happened starting in the early 1970s. In 1973, the APA's Committee on Accreditation incorporated into its criteria for the accreditation of graduate programs and internships specific language prohibiting discrimination of any kind on the basis of sex. Simultaneously, as I will discuss at length below, professional schools of psychology began to proliferate, creating a greater demand for students at both the master's and doctoral levels. Thus both the APA accrediting process and the greater number of training opportunities led to an opening up of the field to greater numbers of women.

Despite the fact that psychiatry recently has been moving away from emphasizing psychotherapy in its residency programs, a proportion of its students continue to be trained to practice psychotherapy. And many of these graduates go on to become psychotherapists, often in conjunction with work as medications consultants and hospital psychiatrists. Therefore, it remains relevant to not only look at women's inroads into the profession of clinical psychology—that field most highly identified with psychotherapy practice—but also to examine their progress in psychiatry. To this end we can see that there has been movement within the profession, but certainly at a pace overshadowed by that in psychology.

At the National Conference on Recruitment into Psychiatry sponsored by the American Psychiatric Association in 1980, the active recruitment of women into the field—specifically the recruitment of female faculty for training programs to provide appropriate role models—was recommended. This recruitment, along with other factors, may be exerting a significant effect insofar as in 1986, women made up 34.9% of all psychiatrists under 35. For psychiatrists aged 35–44, 23.8% were women; for those aged 45–54, 16.9% were women; and for psychiatrists aged 55–64, women represented only 13.3%. Further, in a 1988 survey of graduating medical students conducted by the Association of American Medical Colleges, 47% of those students who chose psychiatry were women (De Titta, Robinowitz, & More, 1991, p. 855).

That women have availed themselves of training in psychotherapy is not surprising given that they traditionally enter any occupation once barriers to their participation are abandoned, as discussed in Chapter 1. But this entrance into the field does not in itself fully describe the feminizing process. Feminization occurs when there is a corresponding departure of men from the ranks of an occupation too. And this is precisely what has happened in the case of psychotherapy. As women have entered the field at increasing rates, men constitute a shrinking proportion of entrants into psychotherapy training programs in both psychiatry and psychology (social work has always been a women's profession). This trend has been particularly dramatic in psychology, where the numbers of graduates at both the master's and doctoral levels have been shooting upward for the past two decades, while the actual number of men has been declining. The Committee on Employment and Human Resources of the APA attributes this shift to men's reluctance to enter psychology at the baccalaureate level. By 1982 women were outpacing men in earning bachelor's degrees in psychology by a ratio of 2:1. This gender imbalance has not been due to any spectacular growth in the number of female graduates at the undergraduate level but rather a real decline in the number of men receiving psychology bachelor of arts degrees (Howard et al., 1986, p. 1321).

While this finding elaborates men's declining participation in psychology, demonstrating that their flight from the field begins at the undergraduate rather than the graduate level, it does not explain that flight. For this, Barbara Ehrenreich's concept of the "yuppie strategy" might be of use. In studying the "new mood" on college campuses in the 1980s, Ehrenreich (1989) states that the

> first element of what might be called the "yuppie strategy" was to choose a college major that corporate recruiters would look favorably upon. . . .

There had been a time when ambitious students saw corporate employment as an option for the intellectually handicapped. Now it was the professions that seemed like a dull, low-paid backwater compared to the brisk world of business.

The choice of a pragmatic, business-oriented major was not always made happily. Many of the college students I talked to in the mid-eighties were suffering from what might be called "premature pragmatism." They were putting aside, at far too early an age, their idealism and intellectual curiosity in favor of economic security, which was increasingly defined as wealth. . . .

With nineteen-year-olds redirecting their energies from sociology to spreadsheets, a negative, self-centered mood settled over the campuses. . . . In 1987, for example, a record 73 percent of students reported "being very well off financially" as their top goal, compared to 39 percent in 1970. (pp. 209–211)

Ehrenreich (1989) points out that the "yuppie strategy" also pervades decisions about graduate training whereby students are "also choosing to avoid the prolonged deprivations associated with graduate study" (p. 210).

The "new mood" that Ehrenreich describes, in which the financial rewards of career options appear to override other concerns, corresponds in time to men's declining interest in psychotherapy as an occupational choice. It is noteworthy that this declining interest also appears to parallel downward trends that are taking place in the occupation. Due to the professional endangerment outlined in the previous chapter, the rewards for choosing psychotherapy as a career may be dwindling. And as discussed in Chapter 1, when men begin to view an occupation as "on the skids," they tend to move out or not enter it in the first place.

Recently professional journals and periodicals have begun addressing psychotherapy's endangerment directly and with considerable concern. Virtually each issue of *Psychotherapy Finances* contains articles such as "A New Managed Care Program Threatens Private Practitioners," and "Is Individual Therapy Being Phased Out?" (i.e., see Vol. 18, No. 8, 1992). More than any other professional publication, it doggedly follows trends relating to psychotherapy's standing at the local, state, and federal levels and its financial health as reflected by a wide variety of indicators. Due to its purely factual style of reporting, any reader can only come away with a troubling sense that the facts speak for themselves: Psychotherapy as an occupation is steadily losing ground in both status and remuneration.

This perspective is echoed elsewhere. "Twenty years ago, the world of therapy seemed like a spacious playing field, with few contenders and almost no losers," writes Mary Sykes Wylie (1992c, p. 30) in the lead story for *The Family Therapy Networker*. At present, however, "the world of private practice seems ominously alive with the rumblings and grumblings of discontent—most of it related in one way or another to money. Therapists worry about where they'll find their next client, and their next paid fee" (p. 30).

"I used to be able to count on regular referrals and clients coming in routinely on a weekly basis," reports Sandra Schrader, a Connecticut therapist.

> But now I see people when they can afford it—which might be for only two or three sessions, or every other week. I'm seeing more people for shorter terms. I'm also finding that the clients I've been working with at all levels of the social strata are losing income, and I'm responding in kind, using a sliding scale with more of them. As far as the future goes, I feel as if I'm holding my breath. (quoted in Wylie, 1992c, pp. 31–32)

In his editorial of March/April 1992, psychologist Richard Simon, editor of *The Family Therapy Networker*, explains that

> these days, private practitioners nervously compare notes about the size of their caseloads and the flow of referrals, and commiserate about the impact new managed health care policies are having on the independence and the income level they have come to expect. They find themselves negotiating with clients about reduced fees, seeing them every two weeks instead of weekly, perhaps ending therapy before the time seems right, wondering how they will be able to keep treating a seriously disturbed person whose insurance benefits will run out after eight meetings. (p. 2)

"Most of the people I know in private practice spend a third of their time drumming up business," reports Jeff Bogdan, a senior clinician with a community health center in New Jersey (quoted in Wylie, 1992c, p. 32). And Richard Wright, director of the Association for the Advancement of Psychology, simply asserts that the "truth is, there are too many therapists. All those people struggling to make a living and working part-time reflect a system that trains too many providers" (quoted in Wylie, 1992c, p. 32).

To support this claim, we need only look at the increase in mental health providers in the 10 years between 1975 and 1985. During that period, psychiatrists increased their numbers by 46%; psychologists by 80%; social workers by 140%, and marriage and family counselors by a shocking 367%. In just one decade, the number of practitioners dispensing mental health services increased over 100% (cited in Robiner, 1991, p. 428).

Psychotherapy clearly appears to be "on the skids," yet women continue to enter the field. As the occupation's fortunes blossomed in the 1960s and 1970s, increasing numbers of women gained access to education and training in psychotherapy. The advent of the freestanding professional school of psychology in 1969, with the founding of the California School of Professional Psychology, facilitated the entry of thousands of women into the field over the course of the next two decades. And because women now constitute a majority of psychotherapy practitioners, it increasingly can be characterized as a "feminine-identified" occupation, to use Christine Williams' (1989) term. As pointed out in Chapter 1, when an occupation becomes feminine-identified, men typically do not want to enter it because it is perceived as requiring "'nonmasculine' character traits—and most men do not want to be considered nonmasculine" (p. 141). As feminization progresses, psychotherapy's connotation as a "motherly" or feminine-identified profession can only serve to stand as a barrier to men's entry, thus exacerbating the process of feminization as men decline to enter the field. Whether or not the practice of psychotherapy has reached what Strober and Arnold (1987) call the "tipping point," as outlined in Chapter 1, is unclear. But what is plain is that men have become increasingly hesitant to make psychotherapy their calling.

In order to better understand men's reluctance to enter psychotherapy training programs, I interviewed a number of men who have made a decision—one way or another—about entering the field. In talking with them about their decisions to enter graduate school in clinical psychology, some of those I interviewed for this book spoke of their apprehension about enrolling in programs that were dominated by female students and/or programs that did not convey sufficient professional status.

Benjamin Turpin is one such man.[3] He is the son of a psychologist and a social worker. He is 26 years old and for a couple of years wrestled with the question of whether he wanted to attend graduate school in clinical psychology after receiving his bachelor's degree in psychology from a major university:

"I really had to figure out what I was doing for myself and what I was doing for my parents. . . . I think psychology is different now than it was for my dad. Well, when he went to graduate school it was kind of an unusual thing, being a clinical psychologist. . . . It was the 1950s and he got lots of job offers. He worked mostly in hospitals and he was always called "doctor," the whole time I was growing up.

"Yeah, it's different now. It's much harder to find a job. . . . I visited a lot of graduate schools when I was home for the summer and I really didn't find them very interesting, professional. . . . Most of the students seemed older, I guess a lot of "returning" women. Everybody calls their professors by their first names. I know that sounds stupid, but for me it means something."

Benjamin decided not to go into clinical psychology because he believes his job prospects would be poor; the profession would not confer sufficient prestige or status, and he would be making the decision based more on allegiance to his par-

[3]This and the following men cited are referred to by pseudonyms. The information reported is based on personal interviews I conducted in 1992.

ents than respect for his own interests. He is now a second year medical student.

"I think medical school teaches you a lot more respect. You give it to your teachers and they give it back. Most of them call me 'Mr. Turpin' and I call them 'Dr. So and So.' . . . The atmosphere is extremely professional. I guess I like being in a medical center where people really are making life and death decisions."

While he claims he is seriously considering specializing in psychiatry, he has recently become quite interested in emergency room medicine.

"I think I probably would do really well in that. I get off on the excitement, that kind of pace. But the pay is really bad, not that psychiatry is exactly great. If I want to make money I should go into surgery. I don't know. We'll see."

For the future Dr. Turpin, status, job opportunity, and pay are clearly issues that have kept him away from the field of clinical psychology. He is a particularly interesting man to interview because he compares the current stature of the field with his impressions of his father's career, begun in the 1950s, a time when clinical psychology was in ascendance as an occupation. He therefore has a vantage point on the profession that most entrants to the field do not.

Bob Rendel is an example of someone for whom the study of clinical psychology is novel. He is 39 and single, the son of a salesman and a housewife. He holds a master's degree in comparative literature and had been working as a carpenter before he entered a professional school of psychology three years ago. In describing the process he went through in deciding to change careers, he reports attending a wine and cheese party that his school has been holding two to three times a year for prospective students:

"Yeah, I was a little surprised that I was the only man there, I mean aside from some of the faculty. . . . My therapist is a man, and I never really thought, 'oh, this is a woman's profession.' But there I was, thinking 'maybe this school isn't really very good if there aren't any men students.' I know I shouldn't think that, but, yeah, the thought crossed my mind."

Bob entered the school despite his misgivings. His own very positive experience in psychotherapy and his dissatisfaction with his work motivated him to change careers. For him being a clinical psychologist conveys a degree of status and professionalism that as a young man he never imagined achieving. His own psychotherapy has convinced him that he can do more with his life than he previously believed. Yet his experience in graduate school has been mixed:

"I love the work. I really do, and I know I made the right decision. But there is definitely a bias against men here."

As one of four men in his class of 35 students, Bob feels isolated and discriminated against.

"There's just a certain attitude in the classroom that men are the enemy. . . . Yes, even when there is a male instructor. I definitely get the feeling that a lot of women who go into this profession have been burned by men—their fathers, their husbands, whatever. Sexual abuse is very hot right now, and I think that since most therapists are women that men are just seen as the enemy."

Bob's closest friend in his class, Marv Levinson, is about the same age and seems to hold many of the same views. He continues to be employed as a school counselor as he works on his doctorate in psychology. He reports that his treatment in a feminizing field can be explained best through a description of a workshop on human sexuality he had to attend to qualify for licensure:

"There were two women teaching the course, and I was the only heterosexual man there. I sat toward the back and just took notes. . . . Then they showed three films of people having sex. The first was of two women—very gentle, lots of touching and fondling. Everybody seemed to like it. The second was of two men, both of them real hunks, and I think everyone in the room found it pretty amazing but didn't really say anything about it because that wouldn't be okay. Then there was the third! [*laughs*] The third was the heterosexual one, ha-ha, and you won't believe what they showed! The man was handicapped from the waist down. Handicapped. And, of course, couldn't get an erection! . . . That's the only way it's okay to show a straight man! Crippled! I just couldn't believe it. So I decided I had to say something to the teachers. But then I thought, 'this will get you nowhere.' Who's going to listen to me? . . . Yeah, that's just how I've dealt with it all along, I just keep things to myself."

For both of these respondents, clinical psychology represents career advancement. Its being a feminizing field does not seem to convey to either of them that it is diminishing in status; although Bob does report wondering initially if the school he was selecting was a poor choice due to the predominance of female students. Nevertheless, both are uncomfortable as men in a women's field. Their complaints are similiar to those of any minority: They feel alternately invisible and denigrated, their experience discounted. They both seem to suggest that heterosexual men are accepted in the field only if they are, in a sense, demasculinized and impotent.

Given their discontent, would they suggest that other men enter the field? Each answered from his own perspective. Bob exclaimed:

"Definitely yes. It's the only way things are going to change. I think if there were more men in classes, they'd [the women students] find out that all men aren't the enemy. . . . It's important to have men therapists. I don't know that I could have made the changes I have if I didn't have a male therapist. I'm not saying I couldn't have done it with a woman, I just don't know. But I do think the option should be there, for men—or really for women also—to have a male therapist. . . . And the way things are going, there aren't exactly going to be a lot of us [male therapists]!"

Marv was more skeptical:

"I don't know. Basically I think it's a good thing for men to have role models, particularly for adolescent boys to be able to come to a male shrink and say it's okay to have emotions and to cry. But there are lots of ways of doing that. Oh, through Big Brothers, school counselors, 12-step programs, maybe even the men's movement. . . . But I don't know what I'd say to somebody who came to me asking me whether or not he should become a clinical psychologist. Maybe at this point I'd say, "go to law school, make a lot of money, and be a Big Brother.'"

The experience of Sean Mather has been quite different from that of Bob and Marv. Sean is 31, the son of a college professor and a designer. He received his Ph.D. in clinical psychology in 1989 from a professional school, did a postdoctoral internship in a hospital's outpatient department, and is now in private practice and studying to be a psychoanalyst.

"It's been completely to my advantage to be a man in this field. In almost every [pre- and postdoctoral] internship I've had, I've been the only man or maybe one of two or three men at the most. It's allowed me to stand out I think. . . . I think in medical school or law school I might have gotten lost in the crowd more, so this has really been good for me. And I like working with women."

Sean acknowledges the downturns in his field and attributes them to an overproduction of psychotherapists more than to women's growing numerical domination of the field. But he clearly believes that talent gets rewarded, and if one is a talented psychotherapist, one can still garner a good deal of status and remuneration:

"I know therapists who are working for $10 an hour, but I also know ones who make $125. I think because it's become so competitive, there are so many therapists competing for the same jobs and the same patients, you've got to stand out. And I think that people with talent can still do pretty well."

Is he doing well?

"Yes, I'd say so. Because I put myself out there. I'm not afraid of speaking up, presenting my work, letting people know I'm smart, I'm a good therapist."

Sean appears to hold a position among his peers opposite to that of Bob and Marv. For reasons that may reside in personality characteristics, class background, attitudes toward women, or perhaps some other variable that is less apparent, Sean has used his uncommonness as a man to set himself apart—and perhaps above—his colleagues. He has used his peculiar status as a socially privleged minority to his advantage. Unlike Bob and Marv who have chosen to keep themselves as invisible as possible, Sean thrives on his exceptionality. He enjoys working with women, does not seem at all threatened by them or their majority status, and perhaps even cultivates their respect and esteem. We can conclude that Sean's career has been enhanced by the feminization of psychotherapy. Due to it, he can be among the elite, whereas in a profession with a smaller percentage of women he "might have gotten lost in the crowd."

Michael Fine represents yet another twist on the question of men in clinical psychology. He has been out of graduate school for 11 years. He is 43, married with two children, and the son of working-class parents. When he earned his Ph.D., he accomplished a feat he had thought he could never reach:

"My father was a baker, an alcoholic, who never went beyond the tenth grade. It was such a big deal that my sister and I went to college, but a Ph.D., no one, including me, thought that that was possible."

Michael has worked as a psychologist in the last remaining community mental health clinic in his city for the past 12 years. He has repeatedly applied to be director of training or chief psychologist during that time, but in each instance was passed over for a woman or a racial minority. He opened a private practice 7 years ago in hopes of increasing his income. At present he works half time as a staff psychologist at the community clinic and about 15 hours a week in private practice.

"Absolutely, if I had to do it over again I would not become a therapist. Things have changed so much just in the past 10 years. It's absolutely a dog-eat-dog environment. I definitely think that because most people in therapy are women, and women want to see women therapists, that men are at a disadvantage."

Michael has struggled to earn an income that he believes befits his training and degree but thus far has been stymied in achieving his goal.

> "My God, I have a doctorate and I'm making less than my brother-in-law [who is a computer programer with only a bachelor's degree]. If I was going into a profession where I was going to invest $40,000 to $50,000 [which is what he paid, but which would probably be twice that amount today], I'd get into something where my future was more secure. I'd go into business, financial planning, something where it's happening today."

And "where it's happening today," curiously enough, appears to be in occupations where women are in a minority.

Such a small number of respondents, selected in a completely unscientific manner, and primarily composed of men who have chosen to enter the field, tells us relatively little about men's attitudes toward the field of psychotherapy in general. These interviews, however, do provide us with some tentative reasons men may be finding training in psychotherapy a less than optimal career choice. What is worthy of note, however, is that for those with negative assessments of the field, none tie those assessments directly or exclusively to feminization. Some of the men do view psychotherapy as "on the skids," but that viewpoint is typically overdetermined. In other words, if women's majority status is seen as a negative attribute of the field, it is tied to other occupational "shortcomings" that men disparage.

This multifaceted understanding parallels my own sense of the role of feminization. If women's growing numerical domination is transforming the field of psychotherapy, it is doing so hand in hand with other fundamental occupational processes that bode significant change for the occupation's practice, status, and organization. I believe, in fact, that feminization cannot be understood apart from these processes, three of which I wish to focus on at length in this chapter.

By examining what I term the deskilling, declassing, and degrading of psychotherapy, I think we can better understand feminization's etiology and long-term consequences.

Deskilling

WILL MANAGED CARE WRECK YOUR PRACTICE?

Dear Therapist,

Many of your colleagues tell us their practices are in trouble. Here are several *real cases* we've heard about in recent calls and letters:

37 hospitals in my area are setting up some form of outpatient mental health treatment facility. My patient load is down 40% in the past three years.

Several PPOs in my suburb are paying therapists $30 a session—and many of my colleagues are taking it. Should I cut fees—or just cut and run? . . .

Hopefully, you're not having problems like these. But if the trend to managed care isn't cutting into your practice you're lucky indeed.

And, what's happened so far is *only the beginning.* . . .

You do have to think seriously about your role in the existing managed care environment—and steps you'll have to take this year and over the next few years to *keep your practice viable.*

That's where *Psychotherapy Finances* comes in. . . . *Now that the rules of the game are getting tougher,* it's more important than ever that you're exposed to every possible idea relating to building your practice and making it more profitable.

(from a direct mail advertising brochure for *Psychotherapy Finances*)

This kind of scare tactic arrives in most psychotherapists' mailboxes with increasing regularity. It speaks directly to the current endangerment of psychotherapy in a provocative and, some might say, exploitative fashion. Yet it acknowledges a process that is altering the most basic character of both psychotherapy practice and professional identity. "Deskilling" is at the heart of psychotherapy's endangerment, and as such underlies the feminization of the field.

In his classic account of the work process, economist Harry Braverman describes how deskilling occurs throughout craft occupations and serves the interests of employers over those of employees (Braverman, 1974). Deskilling is the process by which work requiring the exercise of conceptual and judgmental abilities is separated off from that requiring only routine execution. Braverman shows how it is routine work that absorbs a larger share of employment over time because it permits the substitution of less-experienced, lower-paid workers for higher-paid ones who previously performed the job. Deskilling permits management greater control over the labor process since the individual worker has less autonomy in conceptualizing the labor and in making decisions about the work process. Thus, deskilling involves an erosion of both the substantive complexity of the work itself and the autonomy and control a worker has over the labor process.

Deskilling is a process that is making significant inroads into the field of psychotherapy. The ascent of managed health care and the prediction that it is becoming the dominant paradigm for health care delivery in this country suggest a transformation of the work process akin to that which Braverman applies to craft occupations. The growing popularity of managed care heralds both a decline in the complexity of tasks a mental health practitioner performs and a corresponding reduction in the practitioner's control and autonomy in carrying out those tasks. As full-time private practice becomes increasingly difficult to sustain, due to increased competition, serious reductions in third-party payments, and the upsurge of HMOs and PPOs, growing numbers of psychotherapy practitioners have had to link up with some form of managed care. According to the results of a survey taken by *Psychotherapy Finances* in 1992 (Vol. 17, pp. 1–8), 66% of therapists surveyed had signed contracts with managed care groups, up from 51% the previous year. Forty percent claimed that managed care had reduced their patient load (up from 36%

the previous year); 50% of therapists stated that managed care had reduced their practice income (up from 41% the previous year), and 52% reported that managed care had shortened the length of individual psychotherapies (up from 42% the previous year). Psychologist Mary Sykes Wylie (1992c) notes that "these figures might not be particularly alarming if therapists were not themselves feeling so economically vulnerable to hard times; indeed, many talk as if *they were the health care equivalent of steelworkers*" [italics added] (p. 35).

As psychiatrist William Ayres bluntly informed a group of clinicians in Berkeley recently, "if you decide you're not going to participate in managed care, you can retire" (Herrick Hospital Grand Rounds, June 10, 1991). And in a Distinguished Professional Contributions Award address to the APA, a former president of that organization, Nicholas Cummings (1986), told the following cautionary tale:

> Nobody likes a prophet of doom. I don't want you to say "Nick Cummings thinks we're done for. . . ." But some of us are going to be done in. I recall a colleague in a state that had low HMO penetration. He had a beautiful practice, a Mercedes, and a beautiful home. He was stimulated by his clients; he loved going down to his office every morning, opening it up, and being his own boss. He said to me, "Nick, this will never happen to me." I saw him two months ago, and he said it seemingly happened overnight. "My patients said to me, 'Doctor, I love you, but if I see you, it costs me $80; if I go to the HMO that I now belong to, it's free.'" And he said, "Within three months my practice literally dried up." It will happen to many psychologists because when everyone in an area has signed up to join an HMO or a PPO, psychologists will no longer have a market. (p. 428)

Virtually all forms of managed care significantly erode a clinician's control over the psychotherapy process. They dictate who can be seen, for how long, using what form of treatment. They reimburse or pay a salary only for psychotherapy that they sanction. The clinician certainly has control over the content of the psychotherapy hour, and thus is not precisely analogous to the craft worker Braverman (1976) describes, but the framework in which that hour transpires is one of diminished control and autonomy for the practitioner. According to Mary Sykes Wylie (1992c), "the standards measuring good treatment are increasingly weighted toward brevity, low cost and assembly-line procedures whether they are the most effective or not" (p. 74).

The growth of the HMO also signals a decline in the substantive complexity of the work in which a clinician engages. Frequently the full-time HMO psychotherapist is required to do 36 client hours a week with the hours scheduled for her or him by a receptionist. As one such clinician told me, "I may as well be punching a time clock. Sometimes I feel like a therapy machine. I barely get to know someone, and they're gone." Client turnover is high due to the low number of sessions typically allotted under prepayment plans and the press of waiting lists of people desiring treatment. Since almost no one is seen for more than 20 sessions, the clinician uses the same short-term therapy skills over and over. And according to Jeff Schulman, a Maryland therapist:

> Whatever the client's problem is, it always has to be couched in behavioral terms. In treating a depressed person, you would have to define your goal as, for example, "reducing the number of negative self-statements." Or you say that the client, even one with a severe characterological disorder, is suffering from a "discrete episodic reaction to situational stress," and you promise not to go beyond the immediate crisis that brought him or her into therapy. (quoted in Wylie, 1992c, p. 37)

Perhaps the most illuminating means of understanding how deskilling has affected the practice of psychotherapy is to focus on the history of clinical psychology. For it is in this psychotherapy profession that the deskilling process has had its greatest impact.

In the post-World War II period, clinical psychologists most typically worked in institutional settings performing a variety of tasks—assessment, psychotherapy, research, medical liaison, supervision of other mental health workers, teaching. With deinstitutionalization of first the state mental hospital and then the severe cut backs in community mental health clinics, psychologists increasingly moved into private practice. In this setting, they had virtually complete control over the labor process, but their work typically focused exclusively on the single task of psychotherapy. Private practice, therefore, represented a shift in the relationship between complexity of tasks and autonomy over the labor process. In institutional settings, clinical psychologists performed a variety of tasks but were allowed little control over the performace of those tasks in their roles as salaried employees. In private practice, however, they typically performed only one task—that of psychotherapy—but have had almost total control over their working conditions.

Managed care represents the culmination of the deskilling process. It typically allows the psychologist to engage in the one task of psychotherapy, but it strips her or him of control over the work process and, in the case of the HMO, the workplace. Thus the clinical psychologist of the 21st century probably will once again be a salaried employee with little control over working conditions, but this time around her single function will be psychotherapy, as opposed to the variety of tasks her counterpart performed following World War II. This transformation can be understood further by looking at specific examples of individual clinical psychologists. Through contrasting the work of earlier clinicians with that of more recent doctoral graduates, deskilling of the work in which clinical psychologists engage can be highlighted. What clinicians in the 1990s are doing compared with their counterparts 40 years earlier represents both a decline in the complexity of tasks and a corresponding reduction in control over those tasks.

Margaret Ives serves as an example of a woman who worked as a clinical psychologist beginning in the 1930s and until her retirement in 1973. Ives was born in 1903 and received her Ph.D. in psychology from the University of Michigan in 1938. As she was beginning to write her dissertation she was hired as an associate psychologist at the Henry Ford Hospital in Detroit. Despite the fact that Ives had not yet received her doctorate, given the small pool of psychologists who could work clinically, she was hired to participate

in almost all aspects of the work of the [psychiatry] department except the prescription of drugs.

We saw patients of all ages and in all diagnostic categories,
from babies being placed for adoption to seniles, from normals
to psychotics. I was very glad that I had studied neuroanatomy
in the medical school at Michigan, because I was working very
closely with the neurologists and learned the basics of what is
now known as neuropsychology. Psychotherapy comprised
much of my work in addition to assessment. We went on daily
ward rounds, sat with patients recovering from electroshock
therapy (EST), and took social histories. (There were no social
workers; Henry Ford did not want any.) (quoted in O'Connell
& Russo, 1983, pp. 113–114)

Ives continued to work in this capacity after receiving her
Ph.D., but bristled at the fact that she continued to receive
the same salary because her

lay superintendent said outright that women should not be
paid as much as men and he paid no attention to my chief's
recommendation in this matter.

I received 60 percent of the salary of the male psychologist,
Dr. Schott, and no raise at all when I received my degree. Fur-
thermore, the superintendent's office sent a note saying that
I should continue to punch the time clock because I was a
woman. I refused. I won on the time-clock matter, but not
with regard to salary; so I decided to leave. (quoted in
O'Connell & Russo, 1983, p. 114)

In 1943, Ives was hired as a staff psychologist at Saint
Elizabeths Hospital in Washington, DC.

At first at Saint Elizabeths I taught psychology to the student
nurses, supervised psychology students, and tested maximum
security patients in the John Howard Hall. It was only later
that I did much psychotherapy, first with nurses, later with
patients, especially the forensic patients. I gradually became a
frequent witness in the Federal Court . . .

The psychology branch grew. In 1943, there were two psychologists and two students. When I left in 1973, there were
nearly forty psychologists, many of them doing research under

the auspices of NIMH. (quoted in O'Connel & Russo, 1983, pp. 114–115)

Hilary Westermire received her Ph.D. in 1946.[4] She immediately secured a position at Walter Reed Hospital as a staff psychologist, whereupon she engaged in constructing and administering questionnaires to servicemen regarding the psychological and physiological origins of ulcers. She trained nursing staff, taught psychological assessment, and assessed patients at the hospital. She did not practice psychotherapy as part of her position at Walter Reed, but she opened a private psychotherapy practice in 1962. Four years later she quit her salaried position as staff psychologist and devoted her professional energies exclusively to her private practice:

"At the time [1966], I had more referrals than I knew what to do with. I enjoyed my private practice; it gave me the freedom and flexibility to write, play golf, and see my children more. I could set my own hours and not have to worry about taking time off. . . . I liked being my own boss."

While Westermire states that she missed the variety in the work at Walter Reed, after working there for 20 years, she gladly exchanged that for the autonomy and freedom private practice afforded.

Edith Rosenbaum worked as a school psychologist throughout most of the 1960s. In 1968 she was offered a job as a clinician with a newly constructed community clinic.

"Sure, I had a lot of experience with kids, but I wasn't prepared for this! They needed psychologists and everyone was talking about the shortage [of trained clinicians], so I thought 'okay, I'm up for a challenge.' . . . I worked my tail off; it nearly broke up my marriage I was gone so much. . . . I did everything; no one cared about your 'scope of practice' then. We saw anyone and everyone that came in the door."

[4]This and the following women cited are referred to by pseudonyms. The information reported is based on personal interviews I conducted in 1990 and 1991.

Rosenbaum's position became part time when the children's crisis unit in which she worked was consolidated into another agency in 1979. A year later, she opened a private practice doing psychotherapy with children and families, and in 1984 that practice became Rosenbaum's only professional commitment after the community clinic in which she worked was forced to lay off clinicians due to cutbacks in state funding.

"Of course I like what I do, but I miss the excitement of working with other people. Everyday [at the community clinic] there was a challenge, something new that you had to handle, and it kept you on your toes. . . . Sure, there are challenges [in private practice], but it's not the same. . . . Well, I certainly make more money, but I'm a very people-oriented person, and I miss working as part of a team, solving puzzles, you know, saying 'well, I've never seen this before, so let's figure out together how we're gonna solve it.'"

Female clinical psychologists who have earned their Ph.D.'s in the past decade typically have much different experiences than these three women. First, they have relatively little training in research, assessment, and medicine and far greater training in psychotherapy than their predecessors. Second, instead of being a minority in their graduating classes, they are part of a female majority. Third, given that more than a half of all doctorates in clinical psychology are now awarded to graduates of professional schools (Peterson, 1985), they are much more likely to have graduated from a professional school than a university program. Fourth, it is far less likely that they will be offered positions that allow them to engage in a wide variety of tasks as staff psychologists; there are many fewer jobs available relative to the large pool of clinical psychology graduates. And fifth, most of them envison the exclusive practice of psychotherapy as their professional goal.

Beverly Hammersmith received her Ph.D. from a major state university in 1982. Prior to her graduation, she was already working as a psychotherapist in her capacity as a psychological assistant to a licensed clinical psychologist. After two years, she was licensed as a psychologist and has worked as a private practitioner since that time.

"I love my work. . . . I can totally work my hours around my kids, what they need, what they're doing. I can't imagine a better job for a woman who's interested in being both a mom and a professional. . . . I've had ups and downs in my practice—everyone does, but Rob [her husband] makes enough to carry us through. . . . I've noticed that it is getting harder to get patients, but I think if you stay active, let people know you're out there, you won't have a problem. . . . Well, I've hooked up with one preferred provider outfit, but I really haven't gotten anybody from them; I really don't know how they work, but it's probably a good idea to be a part of one."

Hammersmith was able to establish a private practice before the full effects of federal and state cutbacks in mental health funding impacted local agencies. She receives her referrals from a large network of other clinicians, friends, and acquaintances. She, like the other women psychologists interviewed who graduated within the past decade, entered graduate school with no other ambition than to be a psychotherapist. She has no interest in assessment, and while teaching or research might be "nice," she has never pursued these as professional goals. She also has never applied for a salaried position because private practice has been so congenial to her other major responsibilities as a mother and wife.

Danielle Friedman recieved her Ph.D. from a professional school of psychology in 1986. While she began a private practice prior to graduation as a psychological assistant, she was never able to get more than four or five psychotherapy clients. Upon receiving her Ph.D., she needed to accrue postdoctoral clinical hours in order to sit for the professional licensing exam and to earn an income. She took a postdoctoral position as a staff psychologist for a managed health care, for-profit agency that provides mental health services for a number of medical PPOs. She works 40 hours a week at this job, commuting 2 hours each day. Of her 40 hours, 36 are spent doing psychotherapy. She sees any one individual for three or four sessions on the average. She does not have her own office within the agency.

"I have very little choice in the kind of cases or the amount of cases I see. I wish I had more control but I can see the practical side of managed care. There's pressure to see a lot of cases and some implicit pressure to keep the turnover high, although I've never been criticized for it. If you have an opening, it's filled, so they make sure there's a constant turnover."

Friedman, who is married to an optician and has no children, would like to expand her private practice from its current 7 hours to 20, but she is pessimistic.

"Competition is so great in the Bay Area, I just don't think I'll ever be able to support myself with a private practice— that's just reality. I don't really mind working for [the agency], but I wish I could see people longer term. Sometimes I feel like a robot: 'What brings you to therapy? How long has this been going on? How were you able to handle this before?' I hear there's a computer program where you type in your problems and the 'therapist' responds. Sometimes I feel like that."

Kari Harvey graduated from a professional school in 1989. Because she is not married, nor in a position to receive financial assistance from her parents, she financed her 7 years of graduate school with student loans. Since she was required to take classes and work at least 20 hours a week in unpaid clinical internships, she took out over $80,000 of student loans to pay the $10,000 per year tuition and a portion of the living expenses she amassed between 1982 and 1989. Her one goal is to have a full-time private psychotherapy practice and perhaps become a psychoanalyst, but for now she works 30 hours a week for the mental health reviewing arm of a large insurance company. She is a case manager and as such spends most of her time in a 5 foot by 6 foot cubicle reviewing clinicians' assessments and treatment plans. Her job is to assess whether or not a provider should be able to treat a given client, and if so, for how long and in what form of treatment. She is able to authorize ongoing treatment for no more than 20 sessions.

"It's an acceptable temporary job. I neither love nor hate it. But it doesn't pay enough [$35,000 for full-time work], certainly not for the training I have. I would be infuriated if I had to do this forever. It would be a real waste of my training and my abilities as a clinician. It wouldn't be in any way rewarding or fulfilling as a permanent job over a long period of time. . . . It would feel to me too routine and too bureaucratic. I'd rather address higher-level problems in an immediate, interpersonal way. . . . About 10% of the work requires some careful thought and sometimes some creativity, and the rest [of the time] is fairly routine."

In summary, through the experience of these female clinicians, the history of the deskilling process in clinical psychology is highlighted. Over time, both the complexity of tasks and the control psychologists exert over those tasks has declined. These women's stories serve to demonstrate the chronological shifts in the profession—from Ives in the 1930s and 1940s, who engaged in a wide variety of tasks but had little control over the work process, through Westermire and Rosenbaum, who exchanged variety for control in the 1960s, to Friedman and Harvey, who experience little complexity or control in their managed care settings.

The professional lives of these recent graduates appear to reflect what Carter and Carter (1981) describe in their paper, "Women's Recent Progress in the Professions or, Women Get a Ticket to Ride After the Gravy Train Has Left the Station." In this piece they show that women's representation in the professions has expanded only in those areas undergoing some form of institutional reorganization. After examining women's inroads in dentistry, optometry, osteopathy, medicine, veterinary medicine, and pharmacy, the Carters conclude that:

> It appears that in those occupations in which self-employed professionals have been driven out or bought out and their work reorganized as wage labor, women's employment has grown. Where self-employment has continued as the dominant form of work organization, women's inroads have been insignificant. (p. 493)

Psychotherapy clearly corresponds to the Carters' assessment. As it is reorganized away from the model of private practice to one of "wage labor" or managed care, women's employment has grown. In the case of Danielle Friedman's workplace, two thirds of the staff psychologists are women; for Kari Harvey, all of her fellow case managers are women. Yet in both cases the directors of the organizations are men. Women practitioners are inheriting an occupation that is being deskilled, and they seem to be filling those positions within that occupation that are the most routinized, least complex, and permitting of the most minimal professional control and autonomy. They are making "progress" in terms of increasing their representation within the field of psychotherapy, but due to the process of deskilling, their "ticket to ride" has only been captured "after the gravy train has left the station."

Declassing

Closely associated with the process of deskilling, declassing is also reshaping the field of psychotherapy and appears to interplay with feminization. Declassing occurs when the clientele for an occupation shifts downward in the class hierarchy, thus lowering the image and status of the job (Strober & Arnold, 1987, pp. 130–133). This was illustrated most dramatically in the case of bank telling, as described in Chapter 1. What previously had been an exclusive job serving only a wealthy clientele was transformed into a commonplace occupation ministering to the middle and working classes. Due to this transposition, the public's perception of bank telling diminished. As the class of the typical bank patron fell, so did the public's perception of the status of the employee who waited on that patron. Thus, declassing speaks to the correspondence between the movement downward in the class of an occupation's clientele and that occupation's image and status.

Declassing has been a process that has been evolving for many decades in the field of psychotherapy. The small amount of adult psychotherapy practiced prior to World War II was largely conducted by psychoanalysts or psychoanalytically oriented psychiatrists in either private consulting rooms or small, private hospitals influenced by the "new psychiatry."

In both cases the clientele was predominantly affluent, intellectual, and cosmopolitan. Assessing the patients in his hospital in the late 1930s, William Menninger wrote that they "represent for the most part the upper strata of society, people with broad cultural background and many of them very prominent in their communities" (quoted in Friedman, 1990, p. 77). After reviewing these patients' records, historian Lawrence Friedman (1990) concludes that they were

> very bright. Their intelligence test scores ranged from high average to brilliant, and they had especially strong verbal abilities. . . . Menninger's male patients were usually successful professionals or businessmen. There were even a few prominent movie stars. . . . In most cases, the stock market crash and the Depression had only marginally affected their earning power. Most female patients were married and homemakers. Despite the Depression, they had been able to entertain lavishly. (p. 77)

Following World War II, there was a vast expansion of psychotherapy downward in the class hierarchy. What had previously been the property of an exclusive clientele increasingly was made available to returning veterans and their families, and, over the course of the 1950s, large numbers of the middle classes. As a result of the community mental health movement of the 1960s, not only was psychotherapy made available to the working class but to the unemployed and never employed by the community-based clinics throughout the nation. Over time, the image of psychotherapy as a service for the rich and neurotic, practiced in fashionable Upper East Side consulting rooms, has diminished as all social classes and diagnostic categories have found their way to clinics and private practices sprinkled throughout the urban (and even suburban) landscape. The psychotherapy workplace—often poorly furnished community clinics and HMOs, practitioners' homes, or barely converted residences—carry with them neither the status nor mystique of the high-status medical or law office with its requisite (and typically female) receptionist and support staff.

As increasing numbers of women have opened private practices—some seeing only a handful of clients a week—they have turned parts of their own homes into therapy offices, sublet hours from more full-time clinicians, and found low-rent spaces in apartment buildings and others' homes. Two master's level psychologists practice in the attic of the home of a woman history professor in Berkeley. A social worker with five client hours a week rents the living room of another female social worker, who splits her practice between her living room in San Francisco and a converted back bedroom of her small home in Sonoma, California. A leading feminist theorist and psychoanalyst rents out a basement apartment in lower Manhattan. In order to reach her office, it is necessary to walk through a narrow, windowless kitchen. All of these examples undoubtedly represent inventive, cost-cutting, convenient ways of practicing as psychotherapists. The settings these women have chosen create homelike, intimate, unpretentious working environments. Yet by locating their practices within the private or domestic sphere, a sphere that does not carry the status or authority of the public domain, these clinicians can be viewed as participating in a process of declassing.[5]

In a 1980 study of all licensed clinical psychologists in ten states, Dorken and VandenBos discovered that disabled, unemployed, and blue-collar clients constituted approximately 20% of the clientele for practitioners in private practice and

---

[5]If male clinicians locate their practices in such domestic environments, they too would be participating in this process. But because I have seen nothing published on this subject, I can only rely on my subjective impressions that men do not seem to inhabit offices that are closely linked to the domestic sphere. By way of example, I relocated my private practice from an office building to a converted apartment building that now houses both psychotherapy offices (downstairs) and residential condominiums (upstairs). At my old location, there were an equal number of male and female clinicians. At my present location, there are 14 female practitioners and 2 male practitioners. I realize that this phenomenon, however, does not speak to the tradition within psychoanalysis proper, handed down intact from the 19th century, during which time professionals of all stripes often had consulting rooms in their homes. I would suggest that this ongoing tradition of psychoanalyzing patients in one's home office speaks more to psychoanalysts' consecration of Berggasse 19 and the deification of all things Freudian than to any significant social trend regarding the declassing of the profession.

34% of those who worked as salaried employees. Students and retired people accounted for about 25% of the clientele for private practitioners and 41% for salaried clinicians. Professional and white-collar clients made up roughly 45% of the patients in private practice and a mere 17% of those seeing psychologists who were salaried. By income, less than a quarter of those seen in private practice could be termed affluent, and only about 6% seen by salaried psychologists could be so described (Dorken and VandenBos, 1986, p. 24). Thus, the class and income of psychotherapy patients seem to have shifted downward since the era that William Menninger described.

If the example from other occupations that have experienced a similiar decline can be applied to the field of psychotherapy, declassing then is another component that is interwoven with feminization. If psychotherapy is perceived as less elite than other comparable professional career choices, it follows that men will consider it less attractive, just as many women will see it as an occupational category that is open to them. As the history of bank telling reveals, when an occupation not only experiences deskilling but declassing, the potential for gender resegregation is pronounced.

General Degrading

THERAPIST "GLUT" NO PROBLEM FOR THOSE WHO KNOW HOW TO GET NEW CLIENT REFERRALS

A recent Los Angeles Times article noted that mental health therapists are facing "a market glutted with qualified professionals," a problem of "oversupply," and to survive in their own practices, counselors must "energetically go after business."

Easier said than done, right?

But there's practical, step-by-step help for therapists who want to build successful practices.

(from an advertisement that appears in each issue of *The Family Therapy Networker*)

An oversupply of practitioners in any field certainly would suggest to participants within the occupation, potential entrants to the field, and the public that has awareness of this oversupply that the job category is neither elite nor in sufficient demand to employ all those wishing to participate. The growing supply of psychotherapists in excess of the demand for their services is yet another trend interwoven with that of feminization. It is a process that has arisen due to a complex nexus of historical factors.

As we have seen, following World War II and continuing into the 1970s there was a growing demand for psychotherapists. In response to this demand, educational institutions changed or were created to produce growing numbers of clinicians. Women particularly took advantage of these increased opportunities and have grown into a majority of the student body for psychotherapy training. In the past decade a variety of circumstances, outlined in Chapter 2, have endangered the future of the field. Demand has been affected by the federal government's abdication of the funding of mental health services, decreasing state and local commitment to community treatment, a decline in third-party payments, the rise of managed care, and psychiatry's movement toward more biologically based forms of therapy. In spite of these developments, however, many educational institutions have not altered their training programs. This is most pointedly the case for clinical psychology at both the master's and doctoral levels.

The creation of the freestanding professional schools of psychology revolutionized the training of clinical psychologists. The founding of the California School of Professional Psychology (CSPP) in 1969 ushered in a new method for producing clinical practitioners on an unprecedented scale. Donald Peterson (1985) describes the demand of the 1960s that CSPP's founding spoke to:

> Many scientist–practitioner programs [of psychology within the university] emphasized science so strongly that practice was not only neglected but disparaged. Most programs were tiny. In California, for example, at a time when the general population was increasing rapidly, when California society was in

crisis over rural and urban problems alike, and mental health systems were expanding to proportions never seen before in this country, all the California universities combined were turning out fewer than 20 clinical psychologists per year. The public demand for competent practitioners was strong. The demand from students for access to the profession was growing strident. Demands from practitioners, who faced hopelessly unmanageable case loads, who were dissatisfied with their own training, and who saw no help available from the universities, grew more militant and better organized. . . . The dam was bound to break. (p. 442)

In response to this demand, CSPP inspired the creation of many professional schools, and in California, the creation and expansion of a number of master's levels programs within state and small, private colleges. The response by prospective students was enormous, so that professional psychology programs expanded further, admitting and graduating increasing numbers of clinical psychologists. From the fewer than 20 graduates who earned their doctorates each year in clinical psychology in California in the 1960s, a single campus of CSPP (there are now four) graduated 53 in 1991 alone.

Since the 1949 Boulder Conference that first established the model for training clinical psychologists in the practice of psychotherapy, there has been a 1,100% increase in doctoral degrees granted annually in psychology.[6] And between 1975 and 1985 alone, there was a remarkable 80% increase in licensed psychologists (Robiner, 1991, p. 431).

Supported largely by the tuition of their students, most professional training programs that are accounting for this noteworthy increase have no incentives to decrease the number of students they admit. In order to provide for "administrative costs, library holdings, support systems, and a variety of other expensive services," professional schools seek to maximize their tuition-based revenues (Fox, Kovacs, & Graham, 1985, p. 1044). This situation has resulted in a number

[6]At this rate, it was argued as early as 1951, "the number of psychologists will equal the world population in under 150 years" (quoted in Robiner, 1991, p. 431).

of problems for both the training and practice of clinical psychologists.

First, it has accounted for exorbitantly high tuition. After controlling for inflation, the mean tuition paid by a doctoral level graduate student in psychology increased by almost 200% between 1967 and 1987 (Golding, Lang, Eymard, & Shadish, 1988, p. 1090). Far more graduate education, therefore, is being financed by student loans. In the same period, the mean total amount of outstanding loans, after controlling for inflation, increased 87.8% (Golding et al, 1988, p. 1090). Golding and his colleagues (1988) conclude from these findings "that today's graduate students would think that the current financial situation is less desirable than that of 20 years ago. The loans they are assuming take years to repay and may make entry into a career in psychology less attractive" (pp. 1090–1091).

Thus, both high tuition costs and increasing reliance on loans that burden students long after graduation may make clinical psychology less attractive to prospective entrants who have comparable career opportunities that cost less for training or offer greater remuneration upon completion of that training.

Second, professional schools' need to maintain maximum enrollments has resulted in declining admissions standards over time. James Korn (1984) points out that in 1973, as professional programs were just being created, clinical psychology as a discipline rejected almost 80% of those who applied to its graduate programs (p. 179). Only 9 years later that figure had declined to a 39% rejection rate in graduate programs approved by the APA. For the programs that did not meet the APA's approval criteria—a category in which most professional schools fall—Korn shows that there were almost twice as many places for candidates as applicants (p. 180). A high rate of acceptance insures that many people who were previously denied access to professional training can now participate, and this undoubtedly has facilitated women's entry into clinical psychology. Simultaneously, however, it conveys to the pool of potential applicants and the public in general that the field is not elite, high in status, or difficult to enter. According to William Robiner (1991), vice president of the Minnesota Psychological Association:

> By developing or expanding training programs at a cost of lowering entrance requirements, schools may serve their own needs without adequate regard for the impact of their policies on the profession. High numbers of students or programs might be profitable for schools or faculty, or may help to meet staffing patterns of training institutions that provide clinical services, but might yield adverse long-term effects for practicing psychologists, future graduates, and for the profession. (p. 435)

In a recent survey of 50 master's degree training programs in clinical psychology in California, it was found that most had only minimal criteria for admissions. Only 52% required any kind of minimum grade point average on their applicants' undergraduate records, and of those only 14% required that the cumulative grade point average be at least a "B." Only 34% demanded the Graduate Record Exam (GRE) scores; only 58% conducted interviews with applicants, and only half of the programs surveyed required that applicants have any prerequisite courses. In other words, half of the programs required no background whatsoever in psychology or related disciplines, nor any evidence of showing any particular command of college material insofar as grade point averages were viewed as immaterial (Green, 1990, p. 5). Undoubtedly such admissions standards (or the absence thereof) serve to degrade the field of psychotherapy. If it is perceived that virtually anyone can and does enter psychotherapy training programs, the status of the occupation clearly declines.

This is not to say, however, that students entering these programs are necessarily unqualified, nor that standard admissions criteria such as grade point averages are accurate predictors of who will be a successful practitioner. Undoubtedly gifted clinicians are graduating from professional schools at both the master's and doctoral levels. But because these schools have such mimimal admissions criteria, recruit and advertise heavily to attract students, and accept such a high percentage of those who apply, they perpetuate the perception that anyone except for the "most flagrantly psychotic and grossly inept" can gain admission to their programs (Green, 1990, p. 5). Ultimately this perception can haunt the professional careers of their graduates—mostly women—and serve to degrade the field as a whole. Thus, the many extremely qualified and talented clincians currently graduating from professional schools may be stigmatized by people's awareness of the relatively low standards of the programs in which they were trained.

Finally, the tuition-driven professional school heretofore has remained outside the logic of the market. Founded at a time of high demand for psychotherapists, it has had little incentive to cut back its enrollments despite the decreased demand brought about by the forces outlined in Chapter 2. At a time when third-party payers, employers, government officials, and the institutions of managed care are attempting to contain mental health care services, professional schools of psychology are expanding. William Robiner (1991) cites the state in which he practices as illustrative of this trend:

> Minnesota (a) ranks 3rd in psychologists per capita (is 2.28 standard deviations above the national mean); (b) ranks approximately seventh in the absolute number of psychology licensees but only 21st in population; (c) has had a 191% increase in psychologists per capita since 1976; and (d) dramatically exceeds all known estimates of per capita work force need. Minnesota also has the second highest number of applicants for the Examination for Professional Practice in Psychology. In part, these statistics reflect Minnesota's continued licensing at the master's level. Despite the data, two doctoral-level professional schools have opened in the past 3 years, so there currently are about 500 doctoral-level students in programs of applied psychology. As a result, more psychologists will be trained despite an absence of need. (p. 431)

Robiner (1991) goes on to contrast clinical psychology's inattention to the forces of supply and demand with a similiar situation that developed in dentistry. Due to technological innovations, the success of public health measures such as fluoridation, and the proliferation of dentists, schools accredited by the American Dental Association voluntarily decreased their admissions and enrollments due to employment problems among dentists. Because of an oversaturation of dental practitioners, some universities have closed their dental schools altogether, while others have simply decreased their enrollments by as much as 50% (pp. 433–434).

The training programs Robiner (1991) cites in dentistry are located within universities. Yet in clinical psychology, professional schools account for the majority of graduates at the master's and doctoral levels, and, therefore, these institutions hold the greatest responsibility for the phenomenal growth in the number of psychotherapists attempting to practice today. These institutions should be seriously considering reducing their current levels of training, but because they are solely supported by the tuition of their students, they appear to have little short-term incentive to do so, and in some cases they are actually expanding.[7]

Once they graduate, doctoral level clinical psychologists join forces with social workers, master's level psychologists in some states, and, to a far smaller degree, psychiatrists who still practice as psychotherapists to compete for the few salaried positions in either the public or private sectors. The vast majority of these psychotherapists attempt to support themselves, at least partially, in private practice in the select number of metropolitan centers throughout the country that historically have had sufficient demand to sustain large numbers of private psychotherapy practitioners. But with 65% of these clinicians concentrated in only five metropolitan areas, competition for clients has become extremely fierce (Cummings, 1977, p. 93). In the words of Dorken and Bennett (1986), psychotherapists are becoming "a dime a dozen. . . . Training psychologists essentially as solo-practice psychotherapists is training for technological obsolescence" (p. 383).

[7]A case in point is one professional school that recently moved its campus to more spacious quarters. In order to afford the greater overhead this move entailed, the school cannot admit an incoming class with an enrollment of fewer than 100 students. This one school then can receive at least $1.5 million in tuition from the entering class alone in its first year.

With such a high proportion of clinicians practicing in such a limited number of metropolitan areas, some therapists have erroneously reasoned that an increasing number of clinicians should be trained to practice in underserved areas such as rural communities. But this argument fails to take into consideration practitioners' preferences and intentions. If there exist real shortages of professionals in certain areas, it makes little sense to increase the number of clinicians generally, since only a small proporation will continue to opt to work in underserved areas. In reality most psychotherapists prefer to work in metropolitan areas where residents' high levels of education and income make them likely candidates for practitioners' private practices (Robiner, 1991, p. 436).

Intense competition among clinicians in these populated areas, however, typically drives down wages and status, while at the same time potentially undermining individuals' self-confidence and sense of professional competence and security. This appears to be especially true for new entrants to a field. For new psychotherapists—predominantly women—there can be an enormous sense of personal failure if they do not achieve the status and monetary rewards envisioned as being intrinsic to the field. But what these new practitioners may not recognize is that while they were preparing for and actually engaged in graduate training, enormous changes were taking place in the field they were planning to enter. It was declining due to deskilling, declassing, and general degrading. Carter and Carter (1981) view this as part of a larger phenomenon regarding women's entry into the professions:

The occupations within the census category "professional, technical, and kindred workers" to which women have gained access in recent years no longer have the same meaning in terms of economic or social status that they once possessed. Although they require a fair amount of formal schooling, a large number of these jobs have become low paying, routine, and dead-end—much like other occupations employing large numbers of women. . . . In the seventies, women . . . gained access to many of the more prestigious occupations from which they had been barred before. Yet this access occurred only after control of those occupations had passed out of the hands of

(male) workers and into the hands of managers and bureaucrats. (pp. 500–501)

In keeping with the Carters' general assessment, it
appears that individual psychotherapists are losing control
over their occupation as "managers and bureaucrats" in charge
of governments, insurance carriers, managed care systems,
and graduate schools increasingly determine the direction of
the field. As the model of the self-employed private practitioner gives way to the salaried worker with little professional
autonomy, and as it has become easier and easier to gain
access to graduate training, women continue to enter the field
just as men choose to avoid it. This avoidance in turn can be
related to the processes of deskilling, declassing, and degrading. As discussed in Chapter 1, men choose not to enter an
occupation if it is perceived in any way as being in decline or
"on the skids." In some ways, then, the feminization of psychotherapy, the process by which the field is becoming
increasingly "feminine-identified," can serve to deflect attention away from the fundamental changes taking place in the
field itself, the changes that may make it appear to be an occupation "on the skids." These transformations initially had little
to do with the gender of the practitioners in question, but they
may be exacerbated due to feminization, with the corresponding lower status and remuneration that follow in its wake.
This exacerbation, however, should not be used to disguise
the underlying dynamics that have been outlined. While the
21st-century psychotherapist most likely will be a woman, this
should not blind us to the fact that she will have more in
common occupationally with a wage worker than her professional counterpart in the mid-20th century. As Nicholas
Cummings has pointed out:

> We are now in a revolution around health care in this coun-
> try, which includes mental health care. After being a cottage
> industry for decades—with individual therapists as indepen-
> dent craftspeople—mental health care is now being industri-
> alized, in a vast movement analogous to the Industrial Revo-
> lution of two centuries ago. Eventually, the people who make
> the product—the therapists—will lose control of production,

just as independent workers did when the Industrial Revolution put them all into factories. The control of psychotherapy will shift to the industrialized business interests: there will be five, six, maybe 10 giant corporations that will gobble up all the little ones, and run health care in America—they will thrive on the cheap labor of therapists. (quoted in Wylie, 1992c, pp. 32–33)

And that cheap labor will be provided largely by women.

Psychotherapy with a Different Voice: Feminist Family Therapy

Thus far my focus has been on psychotherapy as an occupation, a job category that is being feminized and deskilled. But of course it is far more than this. In what follows I examine the complex ways in which feminization influences the manner in which human beings are theoretically conceptualized, how psychotherapy is thought to work, what constitutes psychological health, and what the actual practice of psychotherapy looks like.

At first glance it may seem rather easy to perceive the ways in which a greater proportion of women in the field has affected psychotherapeutic theory and theories of technique. Simply put, there is far greater attention to gender today in articles, books, and conferences than there was 10 or 15 years ago. While this reflects the rise of feminism in the late 1960s and its ramifications throughout virtually every part of our society, it also results from the increasing numbers of female clinicians who have made gender an issue in the articles and books they write and read and in the conferences they help plan and attend. In other words, feminism has been carried into the field of psychotherapy largely on the shoulders of its women practitioners, the number of which has been increasing dramatically.[1]

[1]Some, particularly feminist psychologists, might respond to this assertion by arguing that gender is still a marginal category and that even when

By scanning the psychology section of any bookstore or reviewing virtually any journal intended for clinicians, it is impossible not to see books and articles that address issues related to gender and women. This is particularly obvious in the number of journals and books that are specifically feminist. Journals such as the *Journal of Feminist Family Therapy* (founded in 1989) and *Women and Therapy* (founded in 1982) are clinical in focus, while the *Psychology of Women Quarterly* (founded in 1977) contains articles that are clinical, developmental, and social psychological. Due to the presence of journals such as these, articles on women within other journals, and books about women's experience that have appeared increasingly since the mid-1970s, gender has come to be an explicit and salient category of theorizing about psychological development, psychopathology, and clinical practice.

If we look at just three books that some have suggested constitute the "cornerstone" of the new feminist approach to psychology—Jean Baker Miller's *Toward a New Psychology of Women* (1976), Nancy Chodorow's *The Reproduction of Mothering* (1978), and Carol Gilligan's *In a Different Voice* (1982)— we can see the intellectual origins for some tremendous developments in the field: the establishment of a nationally renowned center for the study of the psychology and clinical treatment of women (the Stone Center at Wellesley College); the wide interest in and acceptance of object relations theory among women practitioners; a historically new way of understanding gender differences and why women desire to be mothers; a new means of conceptualizing moral development; and a fundamental challenge to how mental health, maturity, relationship, and autonomy have been seen, not only within the fields of psychotherapy and psychology but in

---

it is evoked or used, it is mostly in nonfeminist ways. Others might claim that the presence of feminists has not corrected or undermined the fact that core theories remain sexist, that even the psychological constructs of the "self" and the "unconscious" are products of androcentric ideology. While not wishing to take issue with these arguments here, I do believe that they downplay the very real advances that feminists have made, despite the fact that they may not be as significant and widespread as many of us would like.

society in general. Additionally these three books alone have inspired literally dozens of others and hundreds of articles and doctoral dissertations (see Kaplan, 1987, p. 17).

Another sign of women's influence on theory construction can be witnessed in the number of women's organizations that sponsor conferences, which in turn account for the presentation of papers written by female practitioners for a female audience. The Association for Women Psychologists, the Feminist Therapy Institute, the Association of Women Psychiatrists, the Women's Institute of the American Orthopsychiatric Association, the Women's Committee of the National Association of Social Workers, and Division 35 of the American Psychological Association (Psychology of Women) are all national organizations that in one way or another promote women's scholarship concerning psychology and psychotherapy. Through their own conferences or through the influence they exert in their disciplines' programs and meetings, these organizations promote women's perspectives. What psychiatrist Marjorie Braude (1987) describes about changes in her field—the least feminized of the psychotherapy professions—can be applied readily to all professional psychotherapy groupings:

> There has been an increase in programs, books and articles by women on issues of concern to women. These have included programs on professional concerns of the woman psychiatrist, gender identity, on rape, battering and incest. . . . There is now a newsletter for women psychiatrists. Women have obtained leadership positions in APA, culminating with Carol Nadelson becoming the first woman president of APA in 1985. She has made a priority of encouraging women to leadership. Above all, there is a dedicated group of women in APA who communicate, support each other on important issues, and have a clear consciousness of women's issues and a developing articulateness and assertiveness about stating them. Their presentations have become an important part of each year's scientific program. (pp. 185–186)

That feminism or a woman-centered perspective has been transmitted into professional psychotherapy organizations via its female practitioners is perhaps best exemplified in the field of family therapy. Here, in addition to numerically dominating the field, women increasingly hold both professional and intellectual positions of power. The president and over half the board of directors of the American Family Therapy Association are women. Authors Peggy Papp, Olga Silverstein, and Cloe Madanes are now as likely to be cited and draw practitioners to their training sessions and paper presentations as such historically significant figures as Carl Whitaker, Salvador Minuchin, and Jay Haley. And according to family therapist Betty Carter (1992): "the feminist critique of family therapy has put the issue of gender unavoidably on the table and profoundly transformed our field. The avalanche of feminist books, articles and chapters on gender topics and so-called 'women's issues' made 'gender' the hot topic of the late '80s" (p. 66).

Family Therapy's "Hot Topic"

In comparison to psychodynamic psychotherapy, which still probably holds the greatest sway in clinical theory and technique, family therapy proper is a relatively new subfield of psychotherapeutic endeavor. Its origins stretch back to the child guidance clinics of the early part of the century, in which social workers attempted to help the families of children who were experiencing psychological distress. As described in Chapter 2, psychiatrists treated the identified patient—the child—while the social worker's role was conceptualized as supportive and secondary. Beginning in the 1950s, however, working with families began to be theorized as a salient, primary form of psychotherapeutic intervention. Still practiced largely by women social workers, "family therapy" as a field unto itself came into being through the theoretical articulation of male psychiatrists and psychoanalysts, such as Nathan Ackerman, Murray Bowen, and Carl Whitaker, who came to believe that individual psychotherapy was necessarily limited and that families were the most appropriate subjects for therapeutic intervention.

Throughout the 1960s and 1970s, these men and others such as Salvador Minuchin and Jay Haley dominated theory building and training within the growing discipline of family therapy. Only one woman, Virginia Satir, reached preeminent status along with these men, so that the usual constellation of plenary speakers at any family therapy conference consisted of five men and Virginia Satir (B. Carter, 1992, p. 69). Despite her stature and inclusion on these panels, at least once as she approached a podium to speak, Satir had to suffer being patted on her rear by Nathan Ackerman, who un-self-consciously blurted out demeaning comments as the audience appreciatively laughed at what seemed to be a "natural" relationship between male and female colleagues.

Throughout its formative years, family therapy fostered the theories of this small number of clinical founders and masters who created varying schools of therapeutic technique. While they were undoubtedly the leaders or "stars" of the field, none was hegemonic in his or her influence. According to Carlos Sluzki, this lack of hegemony has made being a family therapist rough going:

> Imagine going for a voyage on a boat while you are still rebuilding it, arguing with your crew mates whether it should be a motorboat or a sailboat and simultaneously arguing with paying passengers about where your whatever-it-is is going to take them. This metaphor represents more appropriately the crucial challenge of family studies and family therapy: we are at sea, navigating in a rather loosely assembled vessel, and we have to keep on rebuilding it at sea, over and over again questioning our premises, and our premises about premises. (quoted in "The Way We Were," 1992)

Despite the lack of a single, unifying paradigm, systems and structuralist ideas were until quite recently the strongest influences on family therapy. Families were seen as systems with clear organizational patterns that a therapist could and should decipher and map. Far more important than the individual family member was the system of interaction among them that could be altered through therapeutic intervention and instruction. The family therapist stood for clear boundaries, autonomy, responsibility, and, above all, certainty. As veteran family therapist Frank Pittman (1992) wrote:

> Ten years ago . . . the family therapy gurus were mostly straight, white, male psychiatrists. Nathan Ackerman and Don Jackson were dead, but Murray Bowen, Salvador Minuchin, Ivan Boszormenyi-Nagy, Carl Whitaker, Lyman Wynne, etc., were still there with their clear, guiding values, values that were so comfortably agreed on they didn't even have to be spelled out. We believed in staying sane, in staying married, in raising children, in social responsibility. Therapy seemed a vehicle for instilling in people the secure, responsible, emotionally comfortable values of the family we wished we'd grown up in. (p. 58)

Therefore even though techniques and approaches were hotly contested and no "guru" remained unchallenged, the typical family therapist worked throughout most of the 1970s armed with systems and structuralist suppositions and secure in his or her values about how families should be organized and *should* behave.

Toward the end of the 1970s, however, this circumscribed worldview experienced its first fundamental challenge. Writing in the premier family therapy journal, *Family Process*, Rachel Hare-Mustin (cited in Wylie, 1992a) argued that family therapists ignored and, through their practice and technique, denied the fundamental inequality between women and men in the families they treated. "Power aspects of sex roles are largely disregarded or denied. . . . The formulation of dominant mother–ineffectual father as the cause of practically every serious psychological difficulty is made without regard for the underlying inequality that leads to such a situation" (quoted in Wylie, 1992a, p. 22). Hare-Mustin not only challenged the prevailing tendency within family therapy to disparage mothers for being intrusive, distant, domineering, cold, nagging, unresponsive, and/or overprotective but suggested that what therapists considered "healthy" or "functional" families might be truly pathological for women (cited in Wylie, 1992a, p. 22).

Hare-Mustin's was the first salvo of a sustained and

multifaceted critique and campaign to insert a feminist voice into all aspects of family therapy. From the composition of editorial boards to the construction of theories of technique to the adoption of pro-choice stances in professional organizations, women family therapists have made it virtually impossible for clinicians to claim ignorance of gender inequality in their practices or professional dealings. Feminism became such a "hot topic" so quickly that within 7 years of the first published feminist critique of family therapy, Virginia Goldner could write:

> I've sometimes wondered this year [1985] whether feminism has become our newest fashion. . . . I'm pleased, as any outsider wanting to "get in" would be. . . . But . . . I can't help being concerned that the critical edge that is feminism's essential attribute has been blunted by quick success. . . . Taming a dangerous idea by claiming it as one's own is a time-honored political strategy, and I do believe that feminism is dangerous to family therapy. (quoted in "The Way We Were," 1992)

Feminism remained "fashionable" throughout the 1980s, in large part due to the ongoing efforts of women within the field to expand and enhance its influence. In 1984, some 50 women gathered in Stonehenge, Connecticut for "The Women's Conference on Families and Family Therapy" and together discussed ways to increase women's influence in the field. In 1991, another women's family therapy conference— only on an international level—met in Europe with representatives from 30 countries. According to Betty Carter (1992):

> This international meeting was similiar in spirit and agenda to the Stonehenge meeting, which had brought forth the writings and plenaries that had put the feminist critique on the field's national agenda. . . . [By] supporting one another's work, feminists in the United States in the years between 1977 and 1991 were able to keep swimming against the tide: While much of the field delivered "paradoxes," feminists talked straight; while many tried to achieve "neutrality," feminists acknowledged the therapist's value system as a powerful factor; with new models becoming "solution-oriented," feminists have stayed relationship-oriented; while mothers were blamed,

feminists empowered them; as the field asks, "Does it work?," feminists ask, "Does it work for *everyone*?" (p. 69)

Feminist Family Therapy

Despite the fact that books, articles, papers, and panels have been devoted to articulating a feminist perspective on family therapy, this effort remains primarily focused on response and critique rather than proactive theory construction. Upon demonstrating the existence of gender bias in the discourse of traditional family therapy, feminists typically provide extant sociological and political analyses rather than new psychological or social–psychological ones to understand family dynamics. In a recent book on feminist approaches to family therapy, editor Thelma Jean Goodrich (1991) states this most clearly by arguing that family therapists would do well to "stop using our sessions to fix up the people so the system works better and start fixing up the system so the people work better" (p. 8). The two basic strands of feminist thinking seem to be a critique of family therapy for its gender bias and an argument against accommodation to sexist family roles in favor of changing the very nature of those roles in society. According to Betty Carter (1992):

> Feminist family therapy is an attitude, a lens, a body of ideas about gender hierarchy and its impact rather than a specific model of therapy or a grab bag of clinical techniques. Feminists recognize the overriding importance of the power structure in any human system. . . . Changes of heart embraced without a change in the power structure can be rescinded later at the whim of the more powerful member, usually the husband, and can necessitate that adjustments to preserve the relationship be made at the expense of the less powerful one, usually the wife. (pp. 66–67)

Thus, feminist family therapy is typically self-conscious political—attentive to socially constructed power imbalances and interested in altering those imbalances, not merely within the consulting room but, by necessity, in the society at large.

The basic feminist stance toward family therapy is set forth in a book published in 1988 by Thelma Jean Goodrich, Cheryl Rampage, and Barbara Ellman, *Feminist Family Therapy: A Casebook*. The authors clearly state the ways in which they see all elements of family therapy as being in need of transformation from a feminist perspective: "Our thesis is that family therapy has accepted prevailing *gender roles*, ignoring their oppression of women, and accepted a traditional *family model*, ignoring its oppression of women. This failure to notice has resulted in *theory, practice*, and *training* that are oppressive to women" (p. 13).

In focusing on theory, Goodrich and her colleagues (1988) examine the gendered assumptions that are ingredient in virtually all family therapy orientations: Women are and should be the primary caretakers of children; mothers are the source of problems in those children; the "prototypical clinical family" of enmeshed mother and peripherally involved father is ubiquitous; all families are unique and therefore social patterns are irrelevant; "masculine" characteristics are superior to "feminine" ones. Related to the latter, these authors assert: "So much of the literature in family therapy is about getting separate and staying separate, and so little is about getting connected and staying connected" (p. 20).

Ensconced in the fundamental concepts of the commonly adhered to systems perspective are ways of thinking that deny men's power over women. "Complementarity," for instance, "assumes that an observed inequality in an interaction is only temporary and play-acting. At a deeper level of reality, so it goes, the partners are actually equal; they began as equals, will be equal again, and, in fact, will likely switch places in the next unequal power exchange" (Goodrich et al., 1988, p. 16). Further, complementarity suggests that "there is disguised power in helplessness and paradoxical strength in weakness. . . . Under complementarity, the reality of structured oppression is defined out of existence" (p. 17). "Circularity" denies structured power relationships in the same fashion insofar as it "makes everyone equally responsible for everything and no one accountable for anything" (p. 17). The authors exemplify this conundrum by looking at the commonly posed question "does she nag because he drinks or does he drink because she nags?" and the euphemistic term "spousal abuse" (p. 17). Both deny issues of socially constructed patterns of power and control by assuming equality in roles, socialization, and action between men and women. Due to family therapy's insistence upon neutrality and objectivity in all of its theoretical incarnations, feminists have demonstrated that its practitioners have been unable to see its biases and partialities.

This blindness pervades the clinical practice of family therapy as much as its clinical theory. Privileging male clients' efforts over women's, identifying fathers and not mothers as the potential "saviors" of individual family systems, and even talking primarily to wives due to both their greater facility in the "language of feelings" and their awareness of the "subtle nuances of behavior" are frequent occurrences in the practices of clinicians who ignore gender inequalities (see Goodrich et al., 1988, p. 26). This is not to say, however, that feminists offer a comprehensive theory of technique to rectify this kind of practice. "Feminist family therapy is not a set of techniques, but a political and philosophical viewpoint which produces a therapeutic methodology by informing the questions the therapist asks and the understanding the therapist develops" (p. 21).

On the subject of clinical training, however, Goodrich, Rampage, and Ellman (1988) are quite specific. They assert that any training program

> must have women in equal number with men in positions of authority as well as on the training staff. It must have the essential benefits sought in the business world: flexible scheduling, maternity and paternity leave, special supports for single parents and for older women entering the workforce. It must have feminist analysis as the first, not the second, language. . . . We recommend that each supervisor/trainee team have consultants to their process to examine the sexual politics in the dyad. . . . We also recommend that trainees be able to work with both a man and a woman in the role of supervisor at some time during training. (pp. 29, 32–33)

While there is no basis on which to suggest that feminist critiques, reformulations, and recommendations have transformed the theory, practice, and training of family therapy in general, they are widely acknowledged and have entered the mainstream of discussion in the field. It does not seem an exaggeration to assert that feminism is beginning to restructure the theory and practice of family therapy. Feminists are exerting an explicit, prominent, and readily perceivable effect in virtually every journal, conference, professional organization, and public forum that discusses family therapy. And they are "hot."

Professional Hierarchies and the Feminist Consumer

An explicit and highly political form of feminist discourse has entered the field of family therapy rapidly and with wide, although certainly not general, acceptance. This phenomenon can undoubtedly be related to the structure of the field at the time that the feminist movement in the United States was at its most powerful and energetic—the late 1960s through the 1970s. During this time, women social workers were often the typical family therapy practitioners, and male psychiatrists were the typical theorists, writers, and conference leaders. According to Olga Silverstein, now a leader of the field and an outspoken feminist:

> Thirty-five years ago, the originators of the field were all analysts—Ackerman, Bowen, Jackson—and all the theorists were male. But basic workers were women, women social workers. In mental health clinics, the male psychiatrists would see the patient and the social workers would see the family. This got carried over into family therapy. The men did the writing, the presenting, and the women saw the patients. The field had an aura of status which comes in every field where men predominate. Women, however, were really like the nurses in hospitals. When I came into the field about 25 years ago, women got very little of the glory. There were no women leaders ex-

cept for Virginia Satir, and she was treated with a kind of contempt by the male psychiatrists. She had a female take on human problems. She paid attention to feelings, and we use to call her 'touchy-feely.' She didn't have the usual WASP, male, dominant distance. She, however, did have a tremendous following.[2]

This pyramid structure in the professional organization of family therapy—with a small number of male psychiatrists at the top and a large number of female social workers providing clinical services—set the stage for feminist discontent. As women psychotherapists began to be exposed to feminism through political movements and feminist writing outside their field, they had only to look at the unequal organization of their own discipline to recognize the meaning of hierarchy based on gender. As women within family therapy began to write, lecture, and talk informally about the sexism of the field's "gurus" and of these men's concepts and ideas, they did not have to look beyond their own training and their own behavior in their consulting rooms to see that they blamed mothers, denied structural and economic inequalities between husbands and wives, and looked to underinvolved fathers as saviors of individual family systems.

As the work of Jean Baker Miller (1976), Nancy Chodorow (1978), Carol Gilligan (1982), and others filtered out of the academy into the public sphere of feminist discourse, feminist family therapists grained access to ammunition for challenging their field's assumptions that valued autonomy and separateness over relation and connection and that took women's responsibility for child rearing as normal and natural. According to feminist family therapist and author Peggy Papp:

I think the feminists challenged some of the most cherished concepts in the field of family therapy. For example, Bowen's idea of differentiation states that that people who are goal oriented rather than relationship oriented are happier and,

[2]Interview with Olga Silverstein, April 14, 1992.

therefore, he concludes that it's better to be goal oriented. How can you raise children without being relationship oriented? And we pointed out the sexism in some of Minuchin's ideas concerning family structure and organization that often discriminated against women.[3]

While clinicians were being exposed to feminist criticisms of family therapy through discussion with colleagues, articles in professional journals, and presentations in professional meetings, they also were facing a change in their clients, the consumers of psychotherapy. Because these consumers traditionally have been much more likely to be women than men, feminism effected a significant alteration in consumers' willingness to ignore a therapist's gender, or, in many cases, prefer a man. There appears little doubt that requests for female therapists have increased greatly since the early 1970s. And due to these requests, there has been a tremendous growth in the amount of empirical research and theoretical inquiry devoted to the effects of a clinician's gender on therapeutic process and results, a topic I will explore in Chapter 5 (see Goldberger & Evans, 1985; Jones & Zoppel, 1982; Kaplan, 1987; Kirshner, Genack, & Hauser, 1978; Mayer & de Marneffe, 1992; Mogul, 1982; Orlinsky & Howard, 1976; Skolnikoff, 1981).

Marianne Eckardt, who has been in practice since the 1940s, responds to the question of what percentage of her caseload is women, with what has become a common reply:

> Most of the time I'd say two-thirds. The only thing that has changed much in the way people come to me is that there are many more women these last ten or fifteen years that very specifically ask for a woman, and if I don't have any time, they want to be referred to another woman.
>
> In earlier days they would say, "I'd like to work with you," but they had no particular sex preference. Now they feel . . . that they may be better understood by a woman. (quoted in Baruch & Serrano, 1988, p. 292)

[3]Interview with Peggy Papp, April 17, 1992.

Jean Baker Miller has noted this change even more clearly:

> Because of the women's movement, women found more of a voice or sense of empowerment, and women clients wanted to go to women. That was a huge change. Up until a certain point in the late '60s or early '70s, women wanted to go to men because they thought that men were better. If you wanted to go to the best therapist, they thought, you go to a man. Most people wanted to go to men, and I can remember when that started to shift and people started calling, wanting to find a woman. That never existed before. This shift was absolutely related to the rise of the women's movement. So women as consumers of psychotherapy have made a big difference.
>
> Now, male therapists come up to us women and say "can you refer patients to me?" Men who would have never done that in the past. They didn't have to come to women to find patients before the middle to late '70s. They all had their own networks and friends who were referring them patients.[4]

Not only did the consumers of therapy begin to prefer women therapists in many cases, but many of them came to therapy already imbued with a feminist sensibility. Having been members of or exposed to the feminist movement, female clients often were the ones to teach their therapists about gender inequalities and how gendered power dynamics were affecting what was occuring between therapist and client, how sexist assumptions contributed to therapists' assessments and interpretations. Many clients brought with them knowledge they had gleaned from reading feminist theory. Jean Baker Miller recalls how:

> Carol Gilligan's book had an influence on many, many people. I think consumers of therapy spoke to their therapists about the things I said in my book or through the Stone Center [which Miller founded]. And people did that with Carol Gilligan's work too. Ordinary people from all walks of life read her book, and then they told their therapists about what they had read.[4]

[4]Interview with Jean Baker Miller, April 8, 1992.

Author and clinician Jessica Benjamin echoes this understanding:

> Lots of therapists come up to me and tell me that their patients
> talk to them about my work. Then they [the therapists] go
> down to the bookstore to buy my book. Look at the impact of
> Carol Gilligan's book. It had an enormous effect on people.
> Everyone read that book at a certain point. It sold 100,000
> copies by 1987 and exerted a huge impact on people in
> therapy.[5]

For many clinicians this learning process was positive and
enhancing to their work. For others, it was challenging and,
in some cases, threatening. Undoubtedly male practitioners
more readily may have fallen into this latter category.

Often criticized from within their profession by their
feminist colleagues, and often from without by their clients,
male family therapists have in certain ways become an embattled species. Frank Pittman (1992), a longtime family
therapist and psychiatrist, speaks openly about his sense of
embattlement:

> Feminism was a personal challenge. . . . It made us aware that
> we were not all alike; we each were operating under a differ-
> ent set of roles and rules, and we were being influenced by
> forces from the culture.
> But some excruciatingly Politically Correct Feminists con-
> fused statistics with people, confused each man with "all" men,
> each woman with "all" women. . . . They wanted to protect all
> women from all men, as if each man had personally invented
> patriarchy. Some men got testy; we didn't like being seen as
> villains all the time. So we joined the men's movement and
> went out into the woods to beat drums and cry. . . .
> When I read those parts of the feminist literature aimed at
> arousing people into political action, I see how some women
> see men, but I don't find myself and my own experience in
> such nightmares of power-mad men. At an inflammatory
> American Family Therapy Association plenary on violence in
> 1991, one speaker determined that "physically and sexually

[5]Interview with Jessica Benjamin, April 15, 1992.

assaultive men are the norm!" Am I abnormal? (pp. 58, 59, 60)

"Stonewalling Feminism"

Frank Pittman's willingness to expose his disquietude and resentment in print feeds into what Betty Carter (1992) terms a growing tendency to "stonewall feminism":

> I believe we have entered an ambiguous and slippery phase of change—that phase in which the system, having failed to intimidate the upstarts into giving up, now proceeds to water down, coopt and obfuscate the issues. The blurring begins, as always, with language, and so "feminist" becomes "gender sensitive," a men's movement is added to the women's movement, and *voila!* we are no longer talking about *inequality*, but simply about the unfortunate aspects of female socialization on the one hand, and male socialization on the other—the very juxtaposition suggesting an *equal*, though different, set of problems. (p. 66)

Debate about this very issue is loud and vociferous within the family therapy community. In the pages of *The Family Therapy Networker*, psychotherapist James Coyne (1992) responds to Betty Carter by lambasting her as a typical "woman of feminist family therapy" whose "comfort depends upon the disadvantage of other women" (p. 7) and Rhea Almeida and Kenneth Silvestri (1992) deride Frank Pittman's lament about feminism as "a whining farewell to the automatic deference that was once accorded to the 'straight white male'" (p. 8). At a recent family therapy conference, a number of male psychiatrists boycotted the event to protest the large number of women presenting plenary sessions, and men now routinely organize men's discussion groups to counterbalance what is seen by many as feminists' ascendancy in professional family therapy organizations and conferences.

Given this tumult, the direction of family therapy remains unclear. While many speak of stonewalling and backlash in regard to feminist influence, others see feminism's continued growth and ongoing redefinition of the field. There is little doubt, however, that feminism is one of the principal foci of debate on all levels of family therapy discourse. It has achieved this status in part due to family therapy's historical openness to contending approaches. Because there never has been a single "guru" but a plethora of them, family therapy can incorporate continued criticism, rethinking, and debate within its ranks. According to Peggy Papp, "there has always been chaos in the field because there have been numerous competing paradigms. This has always given the field a great deal of flexibility and inventiveness and creativity."[6] Feminism can be accorded widespread attention because family therapists are continually reinventing family therapy, continually "rebuilding it at sea," as Carlos Sluzki has contended, "over and over again questioning our premises, and our premises about premises" (quoted in "The Way We Were," 1992, p. 37).

But feminism also has become an explicit and openly debated perspective within family therapy due to the fact that women have numerically dominated the field while the smaller number of men have controlled it. As Peggy Papp points out, "it's not just the number of women in the field because there have always been more women than men in the field of family therapy. It's the consciousness raising of the women; it's the awareness of the women, the outspokenness of the women."[6] In other words, it is not feminization—the infusion of large numbers of women and the corresponding decline of male participation—that has allowed a feminist voice to become part of the mainstream debate. But rather the feminist movement has empowered the already extant female majority to question and challenge the unequal distribution of power in the field and the gender bias ingredient in its theory and technique. Feminism has been carried into the field of family therapy on the shoulders of its female practitioners. Its influence has been clear, widespread, and explicit. And in this way it stands apart from the other orientations of psychotherapeutic practice that only recently have experienced the feminization of their ranks. It is to what has been

[6]Interview with Peggy Papp, April 17, 1992.

the most predominant and sovereign psychotherapy modality—the psychoanalytic—that we now turn in order to witness the ways in which feminization's effects have been obscured and unrecognized. In this way, the attention to women's voices within the field of family therapy will ser as an important and intriguing source for comparison.

CHAPTER 5

Reupholstering the Couch: Women and the Refashioning of Psychoanalysis

The great question . . . which I have not yet been able to answer, despite my 30 years of research into the feminine soul, is, "What does a woman want?"
—Sigmund Freud

If Freud were alive today, he most likely would be surprised to learn that what increasing numbers of women *want* is to become psychologists, psychiatrists and psychoanalysts.
—Kathleen Hendrix (1992)

Psychoanalysis always has been central to all of psychotherapeutic practice, the paradigm of thought from which all others have emerged, do battle, and measure their success. Due to the early influence of Sigmund Freud on the "new psychiatry," the child guidance movement, and, of course, the practice of psychoanalysis, and because the vast majority of alternative treatment modalities—from Fritz Perls's Gestalt therapy to Salvador Minuchin's family systems approach—were founded by psychoanalysts, psychotherapy in this country has always borne the imprint of Freud's basic developmental theories that privilege the phallus, the Oedipus complex, and the role of the father.

In the past 10 to 15 years this imprinting has begun to be reexamined and rethought. While such theoretical scrutiny and willingness to challenge orthodoxy certainly is not new to the field, up until now it has been the intellectual property of the dissenters and outlaws within psychoanalysis in the United States. From Carl Jung and Sandor Ferenczi to Franz Alexander and Harry Stack Sullivan, men who challenged Freud and his fundamental principles were relegated to the periphery of the discourse and profession in this country. This is not to say that they did not have their own adherents, but once they expressed deviant ideas, they were never accepted by or admitted to the mainstream of the discipline. When referred to within most psychoanalytic institutes or journals, it was in order to convey part of a bygone history without relevance to the present, or as a means of demonstrating a sense of superiority and derision toward those who dared to challenge Freud or his opus.

It seems fairly clear that today this monotheism is falling. It is being challenged in different quarters through varying means and by a wide range of authors. However disparate the language of these writers, their points of agreement are great and their willingness to challenge and revise the most sacrosanct of Freud's tenets has allowed them to effect a genuine paradigm shift that is currently transforming psychodynamic theory and practice.

My purpose in this chapter is to place this paradigm shift in the context of the feminization of the field. I see this as an important goal because the impact of this shift is evident throughout the psychoanalytic world, but the ways in which feminization has been ingredient in this shift have surprisingly gone unnoticed. This is not to say that psychodynamic practitioners are unaware that their field is undergoing a process of gender recomposition, but rather that no one acknowledges the linkage between this and changes in the theory to which these clinicians subscribe. As we shall see, the explicit manner in which women's perspectives have been addressed within the field of family therapy is utterly absent within the worlds of psychoanalysis and psychoanalytic psychotherapy. Yet it is possible that women's increasing participation in the analytic world has effected change that is far deeper and even more global than anything feminists have expressly brought about within the theory or practice of family therapy.

From Drives to Relationships

Within the past decade there has been an explosion of interest in object relations, self psychology, interpersonal psychology, countertransference, and what some have termed the transition from a one-person to a two-person psychology (Modell, 1984). Stephen Mitchell (1988) states this most clearly:

> Psychoanalytic theories of the past several decades have undergone what [Thomas] Kuhn, in his depiction of the evolution of theories in the natural sciences, calls a paradigm shift. The very boundaries around the subject matter of psychoanalysis have been redrawn, and that broad reframing has had profound implications for both theory and clinical practice. *Mind has been redefined from a set of predetermined structures emerging from inside an individual organism to transactional patterns and internal structures derived from an interactive, interpersonal field.* (p. 17)

This shift has refocused theoretical scrutiny from the oedipal to the preoedipal period of development. According to Jessica Benjamin (1988), this

> reorientation has had many repercussions: it has given the mother–child dyad an importance in psychic development rivaling the oedipal triangle, and consequently, it has stimulated a new theoretical construction of individual development. This shift from oedipal to preoedipal—that is, from father to mother—can actually be said to have changed the entire frame of psychoanalytic thinking. (pp. 11–12)

Janet Sayers (1990) is far more blunt and dramatic in her assessment of this transformation.

> Psychoanalysis has been turned upside down. Once patriarchal and phallocentric, it is now almost entirely mother-centered. Its focus has shifted from the past and individual

issues concerning patriarchal power, repression, resistance, knowledge, sex and castration, to the present and interpersonal issues concerning maternal care and its vicissitudes—identification, idealization and envy, deprivation and loss, love and hate, introjection and projection. (p. 3)

However much individual authors might disagree over what to highlight, since the 1970s, psychodynamic theory and practice have been characterized by a shift away from drives to interpersonal relationships, from the goal of autonomy to that of "mature dependence" (Fairbairn) or a "lifelong need for self-objects" (Kohut), from the salience of oedipal to preoedipal phenomena, from countertransference as exception to countertransference as norm, from emphasis on interpretation to a focus on empathy and the real relationship between therapist and patient.

While there are substantive differences among the various authors and schools contributing to this theoretical reshaping, what is striking to me is the similarity of their critique and the correspondence of their reformulations. All share a more relational focus than Freud's in that they conceptualize the basic human condition as one of needing connection to others, rather than mediating biologically based drives that resist human society or civilization. They do not view the oedipal period as the developmental point wherein culture is introduced, but understand the child to be embedded in a social and cultural matrix from birth.[1] Therefore, the developmental picture is reframed so that the preoedipal period is focused upon in contradistinction to Freud's almost unyielding gaze upon the oedipal, the father, and the phallus. This illumination of the preoedipal period leads authors from differing schools to similarly transform clinical technique away from authoritative interpretations (associated with the oedipal father) to the creation of an empathic environment (associated with the preoedipal mother).

[1]The work of Jacques Lacan is not seen as part of this paradigm shift as he has had virtually no influence on *clinical* psychoanalysis in the United States. The appropriation of psychoanalytic theory within academia in this country, however, has been greatly influenced by Lacanian thinking.

By stating rather simply what unites these theorists, I am undoubtedly doing a disservice to the nuances of self psychology, interpersonal psychology, and object relations. But to not acknowledge how much they share in common is to continue the long-standing psychoanalytic tradition of reinventing the wheel and confusing new jargon with new ideas. By hypostatizing the ideas of Heinz Kohut or Donald Winnicott so that their adherents remain unaware of the similarities between self psychology and object relations theory (or the "Middle School" to draw a yet finer distinction), allows the world of psychonanalysis to remain sectarian and surprisingly undynamic. As long as each school publishes its own journals, holds its own conferences, and speaks its own unique dialect, the debates that stimulate and enliven other disciplines are stifled. What remains is each school doing battle with the Freudian legacy in parallel isolation, as though each has developed its critique and reformulation sui generis.

While most psychoanalytic clinicians writing today incorporate some aspect of this paradigm shift into their thinking, few actually acknowledge the range or degree of the transformation, and far fewer still attempt to explain why this shift has occurred. When any explanation is offered as to why theory and technique have been altered, it is most often suggested that because new forms of psychopathology have arisen, new means of understanding and treating such pathology have been required. This has been the premise of Heinz Kohut's self psychology, which he developed as a response to the emergence of narcissism as a relatively new and extremely prevalent form of mental disorder encountered in psychotherapy. Simply put, because the narcissistic personality arises out of faulty empathy in the preoedipal period, not only is a full understanding of that period warranted but a new means of treatment is called for that compensates for the early developmental deficit rather than works through the sort of neurotic conflict seen by Freud in his patients. Today a psychodynamic clinician is far more likely to treat patients who suffer from vague complaints, who feel lifeless and unfulfilled, rather than people who come for help in eradicating specific symptoms, the lifeblood of Freud's practice. Due to this historical shift, it is argued that new ways of understanding and treating are needed, and that the paradigm shift underway simply speaks to this need.

Another explanation occasionally offered for why developmental theory in particular has changed is the claim that new empirical infancy research has brought forth new scientific discoveries that demand alterations in a theory that holds claim to a scientific basis. In this regard, it is the work of Daniel Stern that is most often cited. His work demonstrates that infants begin life not as part of an undifferentiated symbiosis with the mother—a long-held mainstay of psychodynamic thinking—but primed to distinguish themselves from the world of others. Due to this discovery, separation and autonomy do not become the only developmental tasks, as in traditional developmental schemas, but rather connection and interrelatedness—the ability to relate to rather than separate from—also become signs of growth and maturity.

This developmental emphasis on interrelatedness lies at the heart of what Robert Stolorow and others have termed "intersubjectivity," that is, the interface of interacting subjectivities that exists between mother and child, therapist and patient (see Atwood & Stolorow, 1984). Due to human beings' irreducible capacity for engagement with others, the fundamental stance of psychotherapy must be *relational*. And this is precisely the term under which Stephen Mitchell (1988) subsumes object relations, interpersonal theory, and self psychology to describe the paradigm shift in psychoanalysis:

> The relational model within psychoanalysis is a social theory of mind. . . . Freud . . . portrayed the human being with mental content outside of and prior to social experience. For relational-model theorists . . . the individual mind is a *product* of as well as an interactive participant in the cultural, linguistic matrix within which it comes into being. Meaning is not provided a priori, but derives from the relational matrix. (pp. 18–19)

While both the greater prevalence of "self disorders," such as narcissism, and the new infancy research have effected theoretical and technical shifts in psychotherapy, I believe that

they alone do not account for the fundamental transformation toward the "relational model" that has taken place. Given
the scope of the change, I assume that its antecedents are
overdetermined and multifaceted. Therefore, it is important
to focus on those determinants that have been entirely overlooked and are, I will assert, at least as significant as the high
incidence of narcissism and the work of Daniel Stern.

Feminization and many of the correlative phenomena
associated with it can be understood as fundamentally contributing to the paradigmatic shift that has taken place in
psychodynamic theorizing and practice. In fact the very shift
under discussion has corresponded temporally with the dramatic feminization of the field. This is not to suggest any form
of direct causation, but only to point out that the rise of the
"relational model" has gone hand in hand with the rise of
women's numerical domination of the field. While feminization's lasting influence on theory and practice are only
suggestive at this time, three social–historical trends interde-
pendent with feminization seem to have exerted a significant
influence on the paradigmatic shift that has taken place, and
yet they remain unacknowledged by writers in the field. In
this chapter we will look at two of those trends, and in Chapter 6 we will examine the third.

From Shaman to Comforting Friend

In previous chapters, a nexus of trends within the field of
psychotherapy has been shown to account for a diminution
of therapists' authority. Lower status and remuneration,
deskilling and declassing, oversupply and greater competition,
and the ascendance of a biological model both within psychiatry and among the lay public overlap conceptually and
empirically with the feminization of psychotherapy. It thus
can be argued that due to these simultaneously occurring phenomena, therapists may no longer command the same respect
and authority they once did. This may be particularly true for
the psychoanalytically oriented clinician, who, in addition to
most typically not being either a male or a psychiatrist, is an

exponent of a theoretical perspective whose currency has been declining in most departments of psychiatry and psychology on university campuses, and by growing sectors of the population at large.[2]

It seems unlikely then that such significant realignments in the field would fail to impact clinical theory and practice. In fact, the relational model's critique of the classical psychoanalytic stance in therapy may evolve, in part, from such realignments. The tradition of abstinence, detachment, and objectivity as methods of eliciting frustration, anxiety, and insight is founded in an authority relationship between analyst and analysand. The therapist is the unquestioned authority figure who cures by reason of his prestigious training and superior insight. He skillfully identifies and eradicates a patient's resistances through timely and well-articulated interpretations, thus permitting the surfacing of memory and the renunciation of infantile wishes. The relational model therapist, however, eschews such an authority relationship in favor of a "real relationship" between therapist and client. The therapist is a participant in the therapeutic encounter far more than an observer. She not only acknowledges her own countertransference as a normative component of therapy but she utilizes it as a means of deciphering what her client is experiencing. Rather than emphasizing interpretation, she privileges the therapeutic relationship as curative. And that relationship is always collaborative rather than hierarchical in nature.

While the relational model's stance in fact may be superior for working with the self disorders that are the psychopathological hallmarks of our time, and may have arisen precisely in order to work with these disorders, it also may be possible that the relational model assumes the historical diminution of the therapist's authority. In order for a therapist to be accepted as a blank screen who cures through abstinence and interpretation, the therapist must be regarded as an

[2]This stands in marked contrast to the renewed popularity of psychoanalytic thinking within the humanities, where nothing less than a total fascination with both classical Freudian thought and current French psychoanalytic thinkers is de rigueur.

authority whose expertise remains reasonably unquestioned. Because of the trends surrounding feminization, the authority of today's prototypical psychodynamic clinician may not be strong enough to support such unquestioned acceptance. If the public perceives psychotherapy as an occupation that anyone can graduate into, that comes with few of the trappings associated with high-status occupations, and is continually under siege by new discoveries in biological psychiatry that the media herald, then it is possible that when that public enters psychotherapy it will not invest its practitioners with the same authority it may have in the past. While the relational model's technique might better fit today's client, and may simply be a better means of treating people than classical practice, it may also be true that it tacitly incorporates into its tenets the historical decline of therapeutic authority.

Psychoanalyst Arnold Cooper (1990) depicts this decline of authority in his comparison of two Hollywood films that portray psychotherapy. Describing the 1945 film *Spellbound*, Cooper states:

> We were given the picture of the psychoanalyst as the magician who could unfold the mind and discover the dark secrets that are hidden there. That role of the finder of secrets, the holder of arcane special privileged knowledge closely linked with the role of the physician or shaman in society, is no longer the standard role of the psychoanalyst. Currently, the psychoanalyst tends to be viewed as the comforting friend and sharer of knowledge. . . . [In the] recent movie, *sex, lies, and videotape* . . . the therapy session shows patient and therapist sitting on a couch together. The therapy is a shared piece of life, not an interpretive experience. The therapist mirrors the patient's life experience and seems himself to be reasonably seduceable. The earlier movie has its climax in an intrapsychic experience—the discovery of the repressed secret—while the later one has its climax in change through a new experience. All of this could be understood as attuned to our new views of transference and countertransference. (p. 193)

Why the therapist has been transformed from "shaman" to "comforting friend" is obscured if we focus entirely on the move away from drive psychology to the relational model, solely on the history of ideas divorced from their social context. The psychodynamic clinician was more likely to be regarded as a shaman in 1945 in part due to the social realities of his occupational role: He was a man in a predominantly male profession that was accorded high status (Ingrid Bergman's role in *Spellbound* not withstanding). He was most likely a physician who worked in a prestigiously appointed private setting or in a public arena where he was in a position of authority over others. His clientele was educated and drew from the upper classes of society (although this already was changing). Most likely educated in a university, he faced stiff competition in being admitted to and graduating from his postbaccalaureate training program. With insufficient numbers of clinicians practicing, his services were greatly in demand.

In contrast, today's clinician is more likely to be seen as a comforting friend because she is a woman in a predominantly female profession that is accorded declining status. She is most likely a psychologist or social worker who practices in an office that is homelike and unassuming, an HMO, or community clinic. Her clientele can draw from virtually all classes of society. Increasingly she is a graduate of a program with minimal admittance and graduation requirements. And with a oversupply of clinicians similarly trained and eager to provide like services, her possibilities for employment are tenuous.

The Feminization of the Psychotherapeutic Audience

Thus far I have suggested that the relational model may be ascendant due to its ability to speak to contemporary psychopathologies, its reflection of the new infancy research, and its implicit incorporation of therapists' declining authority. A fourth reason may reside in the question of who composes the receptive audience for this model, that is, who is choosing to read and listen to its theorists rather than to those who are more traditionally Freudian.

While it is generally assumed that the relational model heralds a fresh departure from psychoanalytic orthodoxy, I would like to argue that in many ways it is more firmly rooted in psychoanalysis' history and less truly pathbreaking than its various proponents suggest. By looking beyond the new dialects and formats, the relational model represents in a variety of ways the resurrection of past theorists and the importation onto American soil of the work of theorists long deceased.

Stephen Mitchell (1988) identifies Harry Stack Sullivan and W. R. D. Fairbairn as the "purest representatives" of the relational model (p. 18). Both men published their most influential work in the 1940s and 1950s, the former always remaining on the outskirts of mainstream psychoanalytic thought in America and the latter, as a critical follower of Melanie Klein, being virtually unknown to an American audience in his lifetime. As Arnold Cooper (1990) writes:

> In the not-so-distant past it was relatively easy for American psychoanalysts individually, and for the American Psychoanalytic Association organizationally, to dismiss without serious discussion versions of analytic theory that did not fit our preconceptions. "Kleinian" was an epithet rather than a description and the term "object relations" was not part of our vocabulary. (p. 187)

Mitchell (1988) suggests that Donald Winnicott and Heinz Kohut are representative of the next level of "pure" relational theorists. Again, Winnicott's work, as part of the object relations school, was ignored by the American psychodynamic audience until relatively recently. Kohut, on the other hand, began to develop a significant audience after the publication of his *The Analysis of the Self* (1971) and *The Restoration of the Self* (1977). While both of these works represented a fundamental and increasingly explicit departure from classical psychoanalytic thought and presented a new jargon for conceptualizing the mind and clinical work, it can be argued that they bear a striking similarity in substance to the long-discredited ideas of Franz Alexander, Winnicott, and object relations theory in general. Therefore, the "purest" representatives of the relational model are not really new in the truest sense.

Their work, however, has been rediscovered, augmented, and contemporized by theorists such as Stephen Mitchell, Jay Greenberg, Merton Gill, Arnold Goldberg, Irwin Hoffman, Thomas Ogden, Arnold Modell, Robert Stolorow, and others. Basically it resided for 20 to 40 years in Britain, where object relations theory was founded and flourished, and within the confines of the William Alanson White Institute, the bastion of Sullivan's interpersonal psychology.

If the relational model at its core is not entirely new, and in fact finds its "purest" exponents in the work of men whose writings have been available since the 1940s, why then would it suddenly come to ascendancy within the past 10 to 15 years? In addition to the three possible determinants suggested thus far, I would add the fact that there has been a recomposition of the audience for psychodynamic theory. I believe that the feminization of psychotherapy has created an intellectual environment that is more receptive to a picture of human beings and the clinical process that is fundamentally relational. Gender recomposition of the field, therefore, can be seen as one more material reality underlying the paradigmatic shift from classical drive theory to the relational model.

I think the appeal of this model to a feminizing audience can be best understood through contrasting it with the traditional Freudian paradigm. In classical theory, at the center of human development stood the oedipal conflict, with father and son center stage. Females as mothers occupied the murky, uncharted, preverbal terrain of that which led up to the oedipal period and, therefore, did not justify an appellation of its own—hence its designation as simply *pre*oedipal. Females as daughters did not have their own developmental narrative, so their psychological formation was rendered by homology: They too had an oedipal conflict, but since girls were already "castrated," Freud introduced the concept of "penis envy" to account for a girl's turn away from her mother to her father. Even though classical psychoanalytic theory took as its subject matter the preoccupations and concerns of most women's lives—intrafamilial experience, childhood, sexuality, gender difference, and emotional life—many of its theoretical concepts were inhospitable to women—penis envy, women's lesser capacity for sublimation and hence work outside the home, female masochism, and so forth.

The relational model, in contrast, places the mother at the center of the developmental scenario. She is rendered so powerful that fathers and the oedipal period they had dominated are virtually invisible or of far less consequence. Rather than being murky and merely anticipatory or precursory, the preoedipal period is doggedly examined and theorized, and in the work of some, has its own unique stages. By way of example, Thomas Ogden (1989) postulates not only the Kleinian paranoid–schizoid and depressive positions within the preoedipal period but adds the "autistic–contiguous mode," which is "an even more primitive presymbolic, sensory-dominated mode . . . operative from birth that generates the most elemental forms of human experience" (pp. 30, 31). With this kind of attention to charting and scrutinizing preoedipal phenomena, coupled with the deterministic weight with which the mother–child relationship is now invested, Janet Sayers (1990) characterizes the ascendant psychoanalytic paradigm as "mother-centered" (p. 9) and the field in general as "mothering psychoanalysis" (pp. 9, 262):

> The mothering approach to therapy of Winnicott and others is also often preferred because it attends so much more than Freud to the importance of mother-love, and to the all too real effects of its deprivation, loss, and abuse—realities of which Freud seemingly lost sight. . . . Mother-oriented therapy, unlike Freud's theory and therapy, recognizes the very real importance of women in shaping our psychology—not least because of the continuing social assignment to them of childcare, of overseeing the earliest and seemingly most psychologically formative phase of our life. (pp. 10–11)

Chodorow and Contratto (1990) show how what they call "post-Freudian psychology" is dominated by the "fantasy of the perfect mother," who is simultaneously idealized as the potential provider of a perfect "holding environment," to borrow Winnicott's phrase, and blamed for any developmental imperfection in her offspring. The work of Kohut, Stolorow, Ogden, Winnicott, and a host of others who fall under the "relational" rubric presents the mother–child relationship as deterministic. Rather than being undertheorized or undervalued as in classical theory, the role of the mother within the relational model is omnipresent, all powerful, and the cornerstone upon which developmental theory, the etiology of psychopathology, and clinical theory are constructed.

Because mothering and its vicissitudes are understood to play the deterministic role in psychological development, it is the repair or replacement of that mothering function that has come to dominate the relational model's theory of technique. What relational model theorists tend to focus on is not conflict—between the individual and society, or instinctual wishes and superego constraints—but rather deficit and deprivation that result from infantile needs to which a mother inadequately responds. In the hypothetical presence of good enough mothering, a child develops a cohesive sense of self through a series of nonconflictual intersubjective experiences. In the absence of such mothering, development is stymied and pervasive deficits are built into the child's fundamental self structure.

Since psychopathology is characterized in terms of deficit and an unfulfilled need for recognition, mirroring, or holding, as various theorists would term it, psychotherapy becomes the location for filling the deficit. According to Harry Guntrip (1971), a follower of object relations theorists Fairbairn and Winnicott, psychotherapy is

> the provision of the possibility of a genuine, reliable, understanding, and respecting, caring personal relationship in which a human being whose true self has been crushed by the manipulative techniques of those who only wanted to make him "not be a nuisance" to them, can begin at last to feel his own true feelings, and think his own spontaneous thoughts, and find himself to be real. . . .
>
> At the deepest level, psychotherapy is replacement therapy, providing for the patient what the mother failed to provide at the beginning of life. (pp. 182, 191)

From this perspective, interpretations, the traditional lifeblood of classical technique, are seen instrumentally more as a means of conveying understanding and empathy rather than ends in their own right. According to Winnicott, whose work, from Sayers's (1990) point of view, "marks the apotheosis of mothering psychoanalysis" (p. 262), "whenever we understand a patient in a deep way and show that we do so by a correct and well-timed interpretation we are in fact holding the patient, and taking part in a relationship in which the patient is in some degree regressed and dependent" (Winnicott, 1958, p. 261).

Winnicott (1965) concludes that the "analyst will need to be able to play the part of mother to the patient's infant" (p. 163). Thus, the relational model suggests that the real relationship between therapist and patient is potentially curative in itself, providing an attachment to a good object, a holding environment, or a self-object that was inadequate or missing in the early mother–child relationship. If good enough mothering can elicit nonconflictual growth, in its absence, psychotherapy can serve as a corrective developmental experience.

In the recuperation of yet another long-dead analyst whose work fits into neither object relations or interpersonal theory, Axel Hoffer (1991) offers up Sandor Ferenczi as not merely another authority to challenge Freud but as the heretofore missing "mother" of psychoanalysis:

> If Sigmund Freud was the father of psychoanalysis, Sandor Ferenczi was the mother. Psychoanalysis lost its mother through Ferenczi's untimely death of pernicious anaemia in 1933. . . . Psychoanalysis thus became a one-parent child [because] Ferenczi's work on the early dyadic mother–child relationship and its reliving in the analytic situation came to a premature end. (p. 466)

Hoffer (1991) asserts that Ferenczi was psychoanalysis' mother due to his emphasis on the early mother–child relationship and his advocacy of the recapitulation of that relationship within the analytic encounter. In order to achieve this recapitulation, Ferenczi eventually renounced Freud's emphasis on abstinence, privation, and frustration and advocated what he called the "relaxation technique." This involved attempting to gratify a patient's longings in a completely safe, egalitarian environment that was empathic, indulgent, warm, and responsive. In this sense then, Ferenczi's work can now be seen as yet another antecedent to the current paradigm shift.

That female clinicians would be receptive to a theory that privileges the maternal role and conceptualizes the therapeutic encounter in terms of it may be fairly transparent. The relational model moves women from the theoretical periphery to its center, and it conceptualizes clinical practice not only in terms that women can understand intimately but in which they can excel and generally claim experiential authority.

It is clear, however, that redeeming and sanctifying the mother–child relationship as the primary developmental narrative and template for therapeutic intervention has become more than an appealing way of viewing the world for female clinicians. It has become a professional preoccupation, the "hot topic," a chief means of demonstrating that one is no longer chained to the moribund "prison house of psychoanalysis" that is increasingly deemed irrelevant by both dissenters within clinical psychoanalysis and a growing body of clinicians and nonclinicians outside the psychoanalytic orbit (see Goldberg, 1990). Through the rediscovery of ever-greater numbers of male "foremothers" from the annals of psychoanalytic history, and the movement away from interpretation toward holding and empathy, psychoanalytic writers are redefining the discipline along what might be considered "feminine" lines.[3]

From Doing to Being

The relational model not only has rendered the content of psychoanalytic theory more hospitable to women but has fundamentally transformed the goals of the therapeutic encounter in a way that can be more congenial to female clini-

[3]With this assertion I do not wish to suggest that I believe the relational model speaks to some essentialist conceptualization of femininity. I believe that what is regarded as feminine (e.g., being empathic and nurturant) is socially constructed and that the relational model speaks (often unknowingly) to these constructs.

cians (and probably to many men as well). Classical technique emphasized the *activity* of the therapist: His charge was to *overcome* resistances in his patient, *"track down* the libido," and *assert* precise, scientifically crafted interpretations (see Freud, 1912). Freud's metaphor for the clinical mission conjured up a battlefield or hunting ground. The therapist, equipped only with the armamentarium of psychoanalytic theory, was pitted against the tremendous force of transhistorical, universally experienced and biologically based human drives. The patient was a mere vehicle for the expression of these drives, so that the clinician's task was to *uncover* and *unmask* instinctual wishes in an effort to gain the patient's renunciation of them. According to Nina Auerbach (1981), Freud exemplified the "looming man" of the 1890s, who, like Svengali and Dracula, acted as a dark magician who assumed "the virtually limitless powers" of science, myth and magic in order to achieve his ends (pp. 114).[4]

Conversely, the relational model advocates a far different image and intention for clinical work. It prescribes a particular quality of *being* for the therapist. Most importantly, she must *be* empathic. The therapist *allows* for the intersubjective creation of an atmosphere that *permits* the gradual unfolding of the patient's previously thwarted self. There is no hunt, no battle between adversaries waged here. Rather there is a "holding" or "facilitating" *environment* that the clinician *provides* in an effort to establish a corrective developmental experience for her client.

The distinction between *doing* and *being* is one that often characterizes differences between men and women in terms of socially constructed gender identity and sex roles. As Nancy Chodorow, Robert Stoller, Karen Horney, and others have pointed out, male identity is never as secure as that of women; it is something that must be proven and demonstrated continually, "re-earned every day" as Margaret Mead observed (quoted in Chodorow, 1989, p. 33).

[4]It is worthwhile to note that this was what Freud argued for in his theoretical writings on technique. His actual clinical practice, as reflected in his case studies, revealed a more nurturant and less "looming" figure in many instances.

Since it occupies so much of a man's time and constitutes such a large part of who he is in the world, work is a critical arena for the exhibition of "masculine" behavior, the "every day" activity of "re-earning" and reconstructing one's sense of maleness. Through the classical conception of psychotherapy as a sphere for the clinician's activity, maleness can be asserted and confirmed through waging battle with a patient's resistances, through being active rather than passive. Within the relational model, by contrast, the therapist's role is explicitly or implicitly likened to that of a mother. It is a quality of being, a capacity to be *used* by the patient as a container, a holding environment, a mirror. It elicits those characteristics with which women are more likely to be identified—nurturance, empathy, caring, relatedness. As Chodorow (1991) contends:

> Psychoanalysis falls ambivalently between stereotypic masculine and feminine styles, and this dual status has been and continues to be a subject of major debate. In this context, debates about analytic stance beginning with the Freud–Ferenczi split in the 1920s can be read partially as debates about how "feminine" (responsive, empathic, actively present) versus how "masculine" (uninvolved, rationally interpretive, distantly ungratifying) the analyst and analytic interpretations should be. (p. 24)

The classical model well suits a "masculine" way of being in the world through advocating a clinical environment based in the triumph of rationality over irrational, unconscious impulses. If nothing else, the therapeutic encounter is scientific. The process of making the unconscious available to conscious scrutiny is enacted in an atmosphere of neutrality, abstinence, and detachment. The therapist has the mien of the objective scientist, completely separated from the subject he is analyzing. He acts on the basis of reason rather than feeling, observation rather than empathic immersion. He does not proceed in an "intersubjective" manner but objectively, with complete separation between knower and known, therapist and patient, preserving his autonomy, separateness, and distance, qualities often associated with masculinity.

The relational model departs from this rigidly constituted form of science. It posits a fundamental relationship between knower and known. The therapist's primary tool, empathy, mandates a capacity to enter into the other's experience, and this in turn requires a profound level of connectedness and relation. Reason and feeling are not necessarily counterposed, but can be used simultaneously, particularly through the therapist's countertransference. By integrating her understanding of her own internal experience with what she is perceiving in the client, a therapist can make use of intersubjective and interpersonal data to inform her knowledge of a client's intrapsychic life. Above all, psychotherapy is seen as a collaborative effort, not founded in objectivity and detachment, but empathy and engagement. The relational model's understanding of the clinical situation, therefore, corresponds much more readily to what is traditionally thought of as women's ways of being in the world. Not only does it provide a theory that is more hospitable to women but its technique privileges those very qualities of empathy and connectedness that positivist science and classical psychoanalysis traditionally eschew or disregard.

The paradigmatic shift in psychodynamic theory and practice that has occurred within the past 10 to 15 years thus seems to be related to the simultaneous shift in the psychodynamic audience from male to female majorities. That the woman practitioner would be more receptive to the picture of human development and clinical practice painted by the relational model seems fairly clear upon examination. A theory that replaces the "autonomous self" of Freud with the "relational self" of Winnicott, Kohut, and Sullivan as the apotheosis of maturity and mental health can only serve to attract women practitioners who can more readily locate their own experience and that of their predominantly female patients within its precepts.

By claiming this, however, I do not wish to rigidify gender categories nor imply their inevitability. The relational model may also be more welcoming to many men who cannot locate themselves within a paradigm founded on detachment, abstinence, and scientific authority. The very fact that the relational model has been articulated by male theorists not only demonstrates how masculine does not bear an intrinsic relationship to men nor feminine to women but may reveal the oft-noted discomfort many men experience within "masculine" domains. Undoubtedly, part of the relational theorists' critique resides in their personal unease or inability working with traditional drive theory and its attendant technique.

But as much as these men may have been unable to practice optimally within the confines of Freudian dictates, it appears that it is quite common for women to find themselves at odds with that technique. As many authors have pointed out, the traditional psychoanalytic stance has often stood in opposition to both patients' expectations of how women should behave and women practitioners' own expectations of themselves. The work of numerous researchers demonstrates that women in nonnurturant roles are consistently experienced more negatively than men in the same roles. Schachtel (1986) also points out that female analysts are seen by others and by themselves as more withholding when performing their therapeutic role than their male colleagues (p. 250). Similarly, Lisa Gornick (1986) observes that:

> whereas the nonresponsive style of psychoanalytically oriented treatment is consonant with the traditional male role, it is dissonant with expectations that women therapists will be nurturant and emotionally expressive and, consequently, evokes aggressive feelings toward the woman therapist. (p. 262)

Because both patients and therapists alike expect women to be nurturant, gratifying, and emotionally expressive, a professional role that demands abstinence, privation, and frustration is apt to elicit negative responses in patients and some sort of feelings of discomfort and dissonance in female clinicians themselves. Adhering to a model that affords the ability to reconcile gender expectations and professional role would therefore tend to diminish the experience for both patient and therapist of role incongruity. If the psychoanalytic project within psychotherapy becomes identified with mothering, the majority of its practitioners—now being women—will find their work ego syntonic. If patients expect women to be nurturant, their experience of seeing a female therapist who practices within the relational model will confirm many of their expectations. Therefore, the popularity of the relational model, in part, has to reside in its capacity to synchronize women's gender role and work role in the increasingly feminized field of psychodynamic psychotherapy.

The Missing "Masters"

As opposed to family therapy, psychodynamic psychotherapy and psychoanalysis proper have been slow to recognize women's influence. That the shift to the relational model has been effected through its appeal to women clinicians remains unseen within the profession. That women fill the halls when relational theorists speak, clutch copies of Winnicott's and Kohut's work as they travel to their practices, and are the ones who sign up for seminars entitled "The Discovery of the Self in Interaction," "Representations of Motherhood," "Psychotherapy as Negotiation: A Discovery-Oriented View of Psychotherapy Process," and "The Legacy of Sandor Ferenczi: Discovery and Rediscovery,"[5] appears to be taken for granted, unworthy of comment. But a paradigm shift has occurred, and, I believe, it has occurred, in some part because the composition of the audience for this new paradigm has been feminized.

Women's influence in family therapy has been direct and ideological. It comes in the form of explicit feminist criticism and advocacy of attention to sexism and women's ways of knowing. Conversely, within psychodynamic circles, feminism has had very little influence, and women have had an impact more as the *respondents* to new ideas and the resurrection of

---

[5] These were some of the panels offered at the Annual Spring Meeting of the Division 39 of the American Psychological Association (Psychoanalysis) held in Philadelphia in April 1992 that attracted large numbers of women.

old ones than as the *initiators*. They symbolically applaud theories that fit their ways of understanding the world, vote with their feet and their pocketbooks. And because they now constitute a majority, they can throw their weight around and tacitly determine what is popular and what is not. But theirs is not a self-conscious voice within the field in the way that women in family therapy have united and spoken. Due to women's presence and the influence of feminism, there definitely is more attention in psychoanalysis to gender than ever before. But in many ways gender is still seen as a specialty, an area of interest in which women are authorized to speak.

For American psychoanalytic psychotherapists there is no feminist "Women's Project in Family Therapy," no *Journal of Feminist Family Therapy*, no Stonehenge meetings, no Olga Silversteins, Peggy Papps, Betty Carters, Monica McGoldricks, to name but a few. That is, there are no widely recognized women of stature who are explicitly feminist in their writings and teachings and who routinely take their field to task for its failures to attend to women's concerns and needs.

The topics of psychoanalysis and feminism, and psychoanalysis and women have generated a large body of literature in the last 15 years. And there are quite a number of women who now self-consciously identify themselves as "psychoanalytic feminists." Yet these developments have occurred primarily outside of clinical psychoanalysis, in the realm of academia. Within the humanities, and, to a lesser degree, the social sciences, psychoanalysis has been embraced by feminist academicians who routinely use it as a tool for deconstructing texts and investigating how people give meaning to their social experience. Since the subject matter of psychoanalysis is sexuality, childhood, interpersonal relationships, and life within the family, it makes sense that feminists would adopt it for their own purposes and reinterpret or disregard its phallocentrist shortcomings.

Yet the tremendous theoretical developments that have been made within academic psychoanalytic feminism largely remain hidden from clinical practice proper. Rarely is Nancy Chodorow, Jessica Benjamin, Juliet Mitchell, or Jane Flax, for example, referred to in the prestigious psychoanalytic journals. As Benjamin, an academic turned practicing psychoanalyst, describes:

> At the level of conscious thought, feminism has played a minor role in changing psychoanalysis. You seldom find anything cited. Many psychoanalysts have no contact with what is going on in the broader intellectual, academic world. They have no idea of the extent to which psychoanalysis is being used in other disciplines outside of their own province.[6]

When the feminist movement became a major force in American society in the 1970s, family therapy was a treatment modality practiced largely by women who remained virtually powerless within their profession. It was also a field that was composed of competing theoretical and technical orientations, a field that was constantly redefining itself. In other words, conditions were such that a feminist perspective could relatively easily enter the mainstream of family therapy discourse. By contrast, psychodynamic psychotherapy and certainly psychoanalysis were not only dominated by men in positions of authority, they were practiced by them in large numbers. The female clinician was certainly more isolated professionally than her counterpart in family therapy. And perhaps of even greater import, she operated in a theoretical and technical domain encumbered by the omnipresent legacy of Sigmund Freud. As Arnold Goldberg (1990) has noted, "no science was ever born without a parent, but most survive without the continued invoking of parentage" (p. 36). Yet psychoanalysis, unlike any other psychotherapeutic modality and almost any other discipline of secular thought, repeatedly and insistently relies on the invocation of its founder.

Feminist family therapists never had to challenge the divine truth of a deified founder but only had to criticize the comparatively slender output of a handful of mere mortals like Salvador Minuchin and Jay Haley. Feminists' mere presence never constituted a heresy in family therapy. Being a relatively new field with no long-established traditions, fam-

---

[6]Interview with Jessica Benjamin, April 15, 1992.

ily therapy could incorporate even the most blistering feminist indictments without their threatening any monistic belief
system.

In academia, another domain of thought where feminism
has been more accepted, feminists have fundamentally rede-
fined psychoanalysis' tenets. In a review of 12 of the most
recent books on psychoanalysis and feminism, Judith Kegan
Gardiner (1992) reports that "the most startling congruence
among many of the books under review is their concerted
attack on 'the oedipus'" (p. 442). Freud's beliefs that the
Oedipus complex is the cornerstone of civilization and that
fathers, by definition, initiate children into society are psychoanalytic articles of faith that feminists tie directly to male
domination. Through denying Freud's necessary link between
the father and civilization, and focusing on mothers as subjects who actively permit their children's separation and facilitate their entry into the symbolic realm of culture, psychoanalytic feminists challenge Freudian theory at its core.

In the only recently feminized field of psychoanalytic
psychotherapy, where men still hold both theoretical and
organizational seats of power, the kind of direct attack on
hegemonic ways of thinking that has taken place within family
therapy and academic psychoanalysis has not occurred. It
seems as though the field is too brittle and unsure of itself
and/or too fixed and preservative to be able to withstand or
incorporate the kind of assault feminist family therapists have
waged with marked success in their field.

This is not to say, however, that much of the academic
feminist critique has not been echoed within the confines of
clinical psychoanalysis. It, in fact, reverberates throughout the
profession, but often in disguised form. It is explicit in individual articles written on such topics as eating disorders or
the much-maligned issue of penis envy. But it remains only
implicit in the core, contemporary debates. This has meant
that the "attack on 'the oedipus'" and its various corrollaries
has had to come from other quarters, that is, sources that
would be perceived as both more benign and more beholden
to the Freudian legacy than any form of feminism could
present.

Much of the academic feminist critique of psychoanalysis appears reframed in the relational model. Through its rediscovery of some of the great men of psychoanalytic history (along with one woman, Melanie Klein), relational theorists of today can claim a respectable lineage that eventually finds its roots in Freud. Even if it is to recuperate the work of an early dissenter, such as Ferenczi, it can claim a certain historical legitimacy through the invocation of men who were initially Freudians and who always couched their work in reference to psychoanalysis' "father" and his ideas. This sort of deference and "in-house" dissent differs markedly from a feminist perspective that arises from outside the Freudian legacy. American psychoanalytic feminists within the academy have not been compelled to tie their theory construction to Freud in order to disseminate their views in classrooms, journals, and books. They draw heavily from literary theory, sociology, anthropology, and history, that is, fields that have no standing within the insular world of clinical psychoanalysis. Their repeated references to patriarchy, structures of domination, women's desire, maternal discourse, coparenting, the idealization of motherhood, and goals such as "achieving culture without masculine mastery or domination" (Gardiner, 1992, p. 446) not only stand outside the discourse of clinical psychoanalysis but would be seen as nothing less than heretical within it. Even the early work of Nancy Chodorow (1978), which was singularly responsible for introducing object relations theory to a whole generation of feminists and scholars, spoke through the language of sociology and anthropology, aimed to end male dominance, and therefore was rendered invisible within the clinical orbit.

Although it has taken different forms, the centrality of the attack on the oedipus characterizes both the relational model within psychoanalysis and academic feminist appropriations of psychoanalysis. Yet these two discourses remain mutually unaware of each other's existence. The large body of feminist psychoanalytic literature is rarely cited by relational theorists, and vice versa.[7] In the book that most clearly identifies the relational paradigm shift, *Relational Concepts in*

Psychoanalysis, author Stephen Mitchell (1988) has no references to psychoanalytic feminism despite the publication of
a plethora of books and articles that preceded the appearance
of his book by at least a decade. The relational model is both
articulated and perceived as having nothing to do with feminism or the female voice.

Thus, it is possible to surmise that the relational model
has achieved its popularity and acceptance to some degree
through its appeal to the woman clinician and its simultaneous denial of any explicit origins in a woman-centered
epistemology. In other words, many of the same criticisms
academic feminists have made of psychoanalysis have entered
the clinical world, but they entered, in a sense, through the
back door. By embedding the attack on the oedipus in a pantheon of great men such as Ferenczi, Winnicott, and Sullivan,
the relational model has entered psychoanalysis completely
apart from any direct feminist discourse and, in fact, remains
oblivious to the existence of that discourse within the academy. In effect, the relational model theoretically achieves
much of what feminists argue but without directly challenging
male domination and compulsory heterosexuality. Through
privileging the preoedipal, recognizing mothers' subjectivity,
and reinterpreting psychotherapeutic technique as a form of
mothering, the relational model speaks to women's ways of
viewing the world without reference to feminism.

This approach has succeeded in part because female practitioners now constitute the professional audience for psychoanalytic ideas. But unlike the field of family therapy, women
remain largely responsive to these ideas rather than the cre-

[7]The exception to this general rule is the feminists who write for the new
psychoanalytic journal *Psychoanalytic Dialogues: A Journal of Relational Perspectives.* Contributing editors such as Virginia Goldner and Jessica Benjamin uniquely bridge academic and clinical psychoanalytic discourses. The
journal, however, stands outside the mainstream of psychoanalysis proper
and certainly does not command the prestige of journals such as *The Psychoanalytic Quarterly, Journal of the American Psychoanalytic Association, International Journal of Psycho-Analysis,* or the *International Review of Psycho-Analysis,* which define the field.

ators of them. While this appears to be gradually changing, by and large they are not the new theorists; they do not produce and control psychoanalysis' "hot topic" as do women family therapists in their field.

Undoubtedly "theory" in family therapy and psychoanalysis is not truly comparable. For the former, theory tends to be pragmatic, technical, and readily accessible. What jargon exists tends to be easy to decode, and virtually any clinician can apprehend the major debates within the field. Feminist theory in family therapy borrows heavily from an empirically oriented sociology that focuses on gender inequalities, lack of female participation, blaming mothers, men's economic power over women, that is, overt forms of discrimination as they translate into family life, the consulting room, and professional organizations. Psychoanalytic theory, by contrast, tends to be abstract, global, and arcane. Concepts often have multiple meanings and complex histories. In order to fully understand debates within the field, one must have a fair amount of instruction and the capacity and desire to engage with ideas that are often purely symbolic and representational. Because the domain of psychoanalysis is the unconscious, empirical indicators and material proofs are often in short supply. Therefore, to read psychoanalytic theory, much less create it, represents a formidable accomplishment, one that may be more difficult to achieve than in family therapy.

That women can produce psychoanalytic theory, however, is obvious from the clinical history of the field and the activity of feminist scholars within academia today. Helene Deutsch, Karen Horney, Melanie Klein, Anna Freud, and Edith Jacobson, to name only some of the most famous, stand as equals with any of Freud's male disciples. Similarly, the scholarly work of Elizabeth Abel, Jane Flax, Madelon Sprengnether, Nancy Chodorow, and Jessica Benjamin,[8] again to mention only a sample, demonstrates that women psychoanalytic theorists in the academy are writing on a plane at

_____

[8]The latter two no longer can be classified purely as academics since they both have received analytic training after earning their doctorates in sociology and now practice as psychoanalysts.

least equal to the most sophisticated authors in clinical psychoanalysis. Yet there is a shortage of women psychoanalytic theorists writing today for a clinical audience and engaging in the core debates regarding the direction of the discipline. While female practitioners respond to theoretical advances that are in keeping with women's ways of apprehending the world, they typically do not create them.

Psychoanalyst Michele Shackelford (1991) notes this dearth and speculates that it may be due to a number of factors: Women enter the field "as a way of 'helping others,' [and] writing might not necessarily fit in with the accomplishment of that goal" (p. 2). Secondly, "theoretical writing outside the protected domain of academia requires two critical ingredients: time and money," that women professionals often do not have simultaneously due to their typical responsibilities for child care and housework in addition to work outside the home (p. 2).

Jessica Benjamin presents yet another explanation:

> Women in clinical psychology programs aren't being socialized or educated in any way to think of themselves as intellectually autonomous people who have something to contribute to the development of their discipline. They're really being taught to see themselves as journeymen and never thinking that they'll become masters. That's my biggest concern, the anti-intellectualism, anti-creativity in general. The notion that one is learning a practice, a craft rather than an art or an intellectual discipline, is very limiting.[9]

Since, as we have seen, clinical training programs increasingly envision their mission as the production of large numbers of graduates who are trained only to practice psychotherapy, Benjamin may have noted a trend that interfaces with the feminization of the field. As tuition-driven schools with minimal standards educate large numbers of women in the one skill of psychotherapy, female students may not be inculcated with a sense of being part of any intellectual tradition, much less one to which they can actively contribute. Women's capa-

[9]Interview with Jessica Benjamin, April 15, 1992.

city to experience themselves as authoritative, as having the right to participate in the symbolic realm of theory construction, is rarely as accessible as men's. Without the active encouragement of that capacity, it is often extremely difficult for women to identify themselves as intellectuals, writers, and theorists. Since many women seem to be drawn to the practice of psychotherapy as a "helping profession," as one that is an extension of their nurturant activities within the home, it would seem particularly important that such encouragement be available to those women who may yearn for an expanded definition of their professional lives, one which incorporates both helping patients and theoretically conceptualizing that help.

It appears fairly clear that the prototypical psychodynamic psychotherapist is not being trained or socialized to make creative, theoretical, and public contributions to her field. If women within the psychoanalytic orbit do not produce theory and expand the boundaries of their discipline, they will always occupy a lower status than men. That women can create theory has no better evidence than the field of psychoanalysis. But the "great women" theorists of the past can serve to obscure the fact that the vast majority of contributors to clinical psychoanalytic theory, journals, and books today are men. Therefore, it is incumbent on women to begin to see themselves not as mere "journeymen" who effect change as an audience but as "masters" of their discipline, as self-conscious architects of the emerging paradigm within which they work.

CHAPTER 6

Parallel Practice: Psychotherapy and the Contemporary Family

In the previous chapter, two correlates of the feminization of psychotherapy—the decline in the psychotherapist's overall authority and the feminization of the psychotherapeutic audience—were proposed as means of understanding the paradigm shift that has occurred in psychodynamic psychotherapy and psychaoanlysis. In this chapter we will turn our attention to the way the shift to the relational model may also find its origins in the changing social reality of family life that affects child development and psychopathology.

Substantive alterations in theory inevitably bear some relationship to changes in the social environment in which theory construction takes place, although that relationship may not be known or acknowledged. Social dislocations can often serve to make constants into variables and dislodge complacent ways of thinking about the world. If, for instance, family structure is taken to be natural, unchanging, and universal, the social–historical underpinnings of theoretical constructs premised on such family structure may remain obscure. Once, however, the timelessness and uniformity of that family structure is called into question, so too can the theory erected upon its foundations. In keeping with this approach, the rise of the relational model and its preoccupation with preoedipal rather than oedipal phenomena, and with the mother's role in development and clinical practice rather than

the father's, may reflect an implicit, unrecognized incorporation of corresponding changes in American family structure.
The fact that developmental and clinical theory is increasingly
"mother-centered," in part, can be seen as mirroring the ways
in which family life in our society is increasingly mother-
centered. It probably is not accidental that psychodynamic
developmental theory has moved from a triadic focus to a
dyadic one given the steady diminution of fathers' participation and authority in child rearing. Today the likelihood of a
therapist treating a client who never has had contact with any
father figure within the family outweighs the possibility of
encountering a client who grew up in a family similiar to that
of Little Hans or Dora. Yet heretofore the connection between
historical changes within the family and the construction of
clinical theory has remained unacknowledged.

The Absent Father

Over the past two decades American families increasingly
have been characterized by the absence of fathers, through
divorce, separation, or, more than ever, single motherhood
in which a father has never been present. It seems likely that
most psychotherapists have witnessed through their clients' reports the effects of what sociologist Jessie Bernard (1981) calls
the "fall of the good-provider role" and author Barbara
Ehrenreich (1983) has termed "the collapse of the breadwinner
ethic" for men and their concomitant "flight from commitment".

> By the end of the 1970s and the beginning of the 1980s, adult
> manhood was no longer burdened with the automatic expec-
> tation of marriage and breadwinning. The man who postpones
> marriage even into middle age, who avoids women who are
> likely to become financial dependents, who is dedicated to his
> own pleasures, is likely to be found not suspiciously deviant,
> but "healthy". (p. 12)

Bernard (1981) dates the demise of the good-provider
role to the same period and shows how the proportion of
working men with a positive attitude toward marriage

decreased dramatically between 1957 and 1976 from 68% to 39%. During the same period, she points out, working men who found having children "burdensome and restrictive" more than doubled from 25% to 58% (p. 8).

Certainly all the changes in American families during the past two decades cannot be explained away by men's changing attitudes regarding commitment and breadwinning. Economic recomposition, the decline of the family wage, women's labor force participation, shifting sexual and cultural norms, and feminism are critical to understanding how family structure and life have altered. Nevertheless, a crucial fact remains: as the nuclear family disintegrates, it is women who are left with the emotional and economic responsibility for rearing children on their own.

At current rates of increase, it is estimated that two thirds of all first marriages will end in separation or divorce, while today only 9% of American homes fit the breadwinner model where the father supports a housewife and children. Twenty-six percent of all children born in 1988 were born to single women, compared to 18% in 1980 and only 4% in 1950. Currently a quarter of all American children live in a single-parent family. In 1960, only 9% lived with one parent. It is estimated that 60% of all children in the United States will live in a single-parent household at some point before they reach the age of 18. Of these, 89% will live with their mothers; 9% will live with other relatives such as grandmothers; and 2% will live with their fathers. Thus the term "single parent" serves to obscure the fact that "single parents" are typically and overwhelmingly women.

Between 1960 and 1990, female-headed households with children tripled to 25% of all families with children present. It is these households that

> make up a rising share of the poor, soaring from 23.7 percent in 1960 to 53.1 percent of the total number of families living in poverty in 1990.
>
> In 1990, 45 percent of all families with children headed by a single woman were mired in poverty, compared with only 8% of those headed by a married couple. . . .

Even though most single mothers cope heroically, they have less time and money to bestow on their children, making it tougher to help with schoolwork, enforce discipline and otherwise guide their children's development.

National surveys show that children living with a single parent are 62 percent more likely to drop out of high school, three times as likely to be treated for emotional or behavioral problems and more than twice as likely to give birth out of wedlock than are children living with both parents. (Marshall, 1992, p. A-14)

According to Barbara Dafoe Whitehead (1993), "among white families, daughters of single parents are 53% more likely [than those from two-parent families] to marry as teenagers, 111% more likely to have children as teenagers, 164% more likely to have a premarital birth, and 92% more likely to dissolve their own marriages" (p. 62). Additionally, "nationally, more than 70% of all juveniles in state reform institutions come from fatherless homes" (p. 77). Apparently the relationship between crime and single mother families "is so strong that controlling for family configuration erases the relationship between race and crime and between low income and crime" (p. 77).

From 1960 to 1980 the average number of years that men between the ages of 20 and 49 spent in families with young children declined 43% (from 12.34 years in 1960 to 7.0 in 1980) (Furstenberg, 1988). In 1987, 9.4 million women were rearing children whose fathers were not living in the household. This represents an increase of 7% just since 1985, and of almost 100% since 1970. Most women raising children without fathers in the home receive no child support payments. Yet even for women who have been awarded support, 25% do not get the full amount of that support, and 24% receive nothing at all. This, however, represents an improvement since 1985, when more than half of all divorced fathers who were ordered to pay for some part of their children's support failed to meet their financial obligations. Such improvement is not, however, an indicator of fathers' growing concern about their children's welfare but, according to former Health and Human Services Secretary Louis

Sullivan, the result of newly legislated and "vigorous enforcement of child support laws" ("Never-Married Women," 1990).

A study by sociologists Frank Furstenberg and Kathleen Mullan Harris (1990) draws some startling observations from the National Survey of Children, which followed more than 1,000 children from "disrupted" families in a representative sample mirroring the general population in regard to race, geography, income, and education from 1976 through 1987. According to Furstenberg and Mullan Harris, almost half of the children living apart from their fathers had not seen them in the previous year; fewer than half had *ever* been in their father's home, and only a sixth had seen them once a week or more in the previous year. In a typical month, two thirds of the children had no contact with their fathers at all (p. 4).

In a more recent account drawing on the National Survey of Children, Furstenberg and Andrew Cherlin (1991) describe how among children whose parents had been divorced 10 years or more, that is, since they were quite small, only one in ten had weekly contact with their fathers and almost two thirds had no contact with their fathers in the previous year. Since the vast majority of marriages collapse when children are quite young, the authors believe that their "findings provide an especially bleak prognosis for long-term relations between fathers and their offspring. Over time, the vast majority of children will have little or no contact with their fathers" (p. 36). By way of explaining this phenomenon, the authors contend that many fathers simply do not know how to relate to their offspring other than through their wives. Typically, they were secondary parents, less involved in child rearing than their spouses. When they divorce, this secondary or limited role is exacerbated, and, over time, simply breaks down entirely (p. 74).

The absence of the "good-provider role," however, may not only apply to men's literal abandonment of families. As Furstenberg and Cherlin (1991) indicate, fathers' ability to relate to their children only "indirectly" through their wives prior to divorce suggests problematic relations between fathers and children even when they inhabit the same home. After describing how divorced fathers when visiting their children behave "more like close relatives than parents," Furstenberg and Cherlin quickly point out that they are not certain that fathers in intact families are any more involved with their children than the nonresidential fathers they studied. In fact, the children of divorce who had at least some contact with their fathers were only slightly less likely than the children of intact families to report that they frequently did things with their fathers or spent as much time with them as they would have liked (p. 36). "'Father absence,' far from a social aberration or an individual pathology is virtually a foregone conclusion, 'normal' American family life," notes Judith Levine in *My Enemy, My Love: Man-hating and Ambivalence in Women's Lives* (1992, p. 191). And that absence can exist even though fathers may be physically present but emotionally unavailable, passive, uninterested, and/or unable to connect.

Far worse than normative father absence, however, is the way the "fall of the good-provider role" may also speak to the sexual and physical abuse perpetrated by adult males against adult women and minor females and males within the family. Although it is difficult to know with any precision how much violence occurs within families, studies show that about one in four women are physically abused by their husbands or male partners. Almost a quarter of adults report having been sexually abused as children. Two thirds of the victims were girls, and over 90% of their abusers were adult men. Of these adult men, almost a quarter were male relatives. While the absence of historical data makes it impossible to say whether or not these figures represent a change in the incidence of family violence, reporting of abuse has steadily increased over the past decade.

Feminist author Sara Ruddick (1990) looks at these sorts of data and offers one kind of conclusion that undoubtedly makes sense to many people, particularly those who have suffered abuse within their families:

> What is striking is the extent and variety of the psychological, sexual, and physical battery suffered by women and children of all classes and social groups, often (though by no means always) at the hands of fathers, their mothers' male lovers, or male relatives.

If putative fathers are absent or perpetually disappearing and actual fathers are controlling or abusive, who needs a father? What mother would want to live with one or wish one on her children? Even social theorists who bewail the toll of divorce and the immiseration of female-headed households recognize that while a good father is good for his children, a bad father is worse than none at all. (p. 224)

Given this very cursory review of current trends regarding family life, it appears clear that men's role in the family is undergoing a significant shift. As divorce, separation, and out of wedlock births rise, fathers are increasingly shirking their previously socially sanctioned roles as breadwinners, authority figures, and moral guides by means of literal abandonment of their families or by violation of these roles through physical and sexual abuse of their children. While there are definite and significant exceptions to this trend—particularly among professional and highly educated men who seem to increasingly value their involvement in their children's lives—overall, more and more women and children are being confronted with life *without* father. This is not to say that women as mothers are not figures of authority to their children, nor that fathers in reality have always or even typically acted as moral guides or authority figures. Rather, a smaller percentage of men are actually occupying the father's role in our society than in any time in recent history, and the ideal typical set of expectations that previously accompanied that role have increasingly been abandoned by adult men.[1]

As men leave or have never been involved with their families of procreation, and women are compelled to provide

[1]There are some authors who would dispute this analysis by suggesting that while rates of divorce and single motherhood have never been higher, fathers previously left families through death and abandonment. Due to shorter life expectancies, children often grew up in single-parent households prior to the 20th century. While this debate is outside the scope of my concerns here, I can only suggest that this purely demographic argument sidesteps any discussion of meaning, psychology, and values. A father's death does not contradict "the good-provider role," nor does it have the same meaning—on his children's intrapsychic life or for culturally held values—as his divorce and concomitant abandonment of his children.

materially and emotionally for themselves and their children (or grandchildren), the field of psychotherapy seems to mimic—on a professional level—a similar transformation. While there is no evidence that men are leaving the field, it is clear they are entering at rates so small that psychotherapy is decidedly on its way to becoming a women's occupation. Thus, as adult clients come to therapy searching for help in repairing the injuries originating in their families of origin, and as children and adolescents come looking for assistance in struggling with their current family problems, increasingly they will encounter the same situation with which so many of them are all too familiar, namely, a world without men. This is not to suggest that many clients will have had literally no contact with adult men. But many have and will increasingly have little sustained contact with father figures who play an actively supportive and caring role in their lives. Because children living without both parents are three times more likely to be "treated for emotional or behavioral problems" than children living with both parents, and because women are overwhelmingly the single parents in our society, it is quite likely that one form or another of father hunger will be seen in clinicians' consulting rooms. And if current trends continue, father absence will increasingly play a role in people's lives and thus in psychotherapy.

The Vanishing Male Therapist

Due to the feminization of psychotherapy, the experience of examining one's inner life by working with a caring and authoritative male therapist is becoming less common and may soon be anachronous. Men who ideally could serve as benign, caring, and attentive figures of authority—a role increasingly left vacant in families today—represent a small minority in most clinical training programs throughout the country. Therefore, a major helping profession, one that traditionally has served to counterbalance the effects of pathological aspects of family and society, is in the process of becoming yet another arena of life—like the day-care center and the school—where adult men are in short supply. While this may be a welcomed relief to potential clients who have been abused or neglected by men, it also serves to confirm the idea—rightly or wrongly—that men are not available to turn to for help with emotional and psychological problems.

For people raised without fathers or with ones who are only remotely involved, the field of psychotherapy increasingly replicates the terrain of family life. If the feminization of other occupations can serve as a guide, we can expect that men will continue to have a particular type of continuing presence in the field—namely as remotely involved administrators, teachers, supervisors, and theorists and as psychiatrists providing medications consults and hospital care. But the hands-on, day-to-day work of psychotherapy increasingly will be the work of women alone. For the more than 50% of American children who will live at some point before age 18 in a single-woman household, the experience of psychotherapy, if they choose to have it, might appear quite familiar: Men may come and go—as psychiatrists offering a quick fix through medications; as supervisors, administrators, and teachers who have some imperceptible control or influence over their female therapists—but women are the ones who remain constant in their attention, willing to focus their interest and understanding on the intimate, dirty, and mundane details of people's lives.

Until relatively recently it was almost universally asserted in the psychodynamic literature that the sex of the therapist was inconsequential: Patients developed a transference neurosis according to the dynamics of their own unconscious fantasies that were little affected by the actual attributes of their therapist. In many ways this fiction could prevail as long as the gender of the therapist remained male and that of the patient remained female: "Because the dominant narrative of a male doctor treating a woman patient maintains the normative structure of men occupying postions of authority over women, the importance of the gender of the participants in the therapeutic dialogue is obscured" (Gornick, 1986, p. 258).

More recently as this "dominant narrative" has altered,

the gender of the therapist has been recognized as being an important variable in the therapeutic interplay between internal and external forces. While the therapist's sex is now generally thought to have some role in influencing the nature of the transference in most psychotherapies, in many instances, therapist's gender has become a significant focus of clinical theory. A number of authors argue that a therapist's sex often should be the basis of referral in cases of early parental loss, incest, certain borderline pathologies, sexual abuse, gender identity confusion, sexual disorders, certain instances of paranoia in men, and second therapies in which "therapists of different sex might permit the evocation of different conflicts within the same patient regardless of the technical abilities or dynamic understanding of one therapist or the other" (Skolnikoff, 1981, p. 14).

Yet, as clinical theory becomes more sensitized to the issue of therapist's gender and the role it can effect in the choice of therapist and the course of therapy, the realities of the field increasingly undermine gender as being a salient clinical issue. The sex of the therapist is of particular interest as long as there is the option or choice of having a male or female therapist, as long as gender is a variable rather than a constant. Due to feminization, however, the variable of therapist's sex is being transformed into a constant. What this means for actual clinical practice is that therapists will have one less option for therapeutic intervention. In other words, a debate about whether it is best for a client clinically to see a female or male therapist is being rendered superfluous due to the declining presence of men in the field.

To some the increasing absence of male psychotherapists will only serve to confirm the belief that men are uninterested in occupying nurturant roles, in promoting emotional connection and growth through the work they do. To others it will signal relief. If men in positions of authority are viewed as potential abusers and betrayers, their departure from the field of psychotherapy removes the potential for that mistreatment. One clear example of this lies in the issue of male therapists' sexual abuse of their patients. Increasingly the media have focused attention on clinicians' sexual misconduct, and it is the male psychotherapist who is overwhelming responsible for the abuse reported. A series of articles written in 1991 in the *San Francisco Examiner* entitled "Doctors of Desire" declares

> an epidemic of sexual misconduct plaguing up to 12% of the consulting rooms in the state [California] where male psychotherapists practice. . . .
>
> National surveys have found that male practitioners are involved 85 to 96% of the time. While adult heterosexual advances easily predominate, there are child molestations and homosexual seductions as well. It is rarely the case, however, that a female therapist has sex with her male patient. (p. A-18)

In studies of practicing psychiatrists and psychologists, it has been found that about 10% of the male respondents admit to having sexual contact with their patients (see Holroyd & Brodsky, 1977). In one study of male and female psychologists, 8.1% of the men and 1% of the female practitioners admitted to having actual intercourse with current or past patients, and a "significantly higher proportion of males than females believed that erotic contact with patients might be beneficial to their treatment" (Holroyd & Brodsky, 1977, p. 847). For a number of reasons, it is highly likely that the figures on practitioner sexual misconduct are conservative, that is, that they understate the case: It is widely known that sexual contact between patient and therapist is unethical (and in some states, illegal); studies of clinicians' sexual misconduct are based on self-report; in the studies cited, anywhere between 30% and 54% of those therapists sent questionnaires fail to return them. Nevertheless, at least one firm conclusion can be drawn from the surveys that have been conducted: "Erotic contact and intercourse are almost always between male therapists and female clients" (Holroyd & Brodsky, 1977, p. 848).

Having cited this, it is important to point out that even the most liberal estimates indicate that only a small minority of male psychotherapists sexually abuse their patients. But for those who are already suspicious of the intentions and motivations of male authority figures, studies of sexual misconduct in the consulting room and the media's reporting of them will only serve to confirm that men's departure from the field as a result of feminization is a positive development. Many could argue that Ruddick's (1990) conclusion about the family, "while a good father is good for his children, a bad father is worse than none at all" (p. 224) applies to psychotherapy as well. While it is beneficial for the field to have good male clinicians, it is better to offer none at all rather than ones who could potentially inflict harm, particularly to their female clients who have turned to them for repair and help.

Further, since it is estimated that roughly two thirds of outpatient psychotherapy clients are female, feminization also may make the field seem even less hospitable to the prospective male client. It has been shown that a man's fear of identifying with a female therapist can inhibit his willingness to work in psychotherapy with a woman (Goldberger & Evans, 1985). Such a fear is believed to be particularly salient for more disturbed male clients, whose uncertainty about their own identity renders identification with a female therapist particularly threatening (Goldberger & Evans, 1985; Mogul, 1982). But as Stoller (1974) and Mead (cited in Chodorow, 1989) have pointed out, even "normal" masculinity requires daily "re-earning" and continual environmental support. Therefore, merely entering into the increasingly feminine-identified domain of psychotherapy may be somewhat challenging to men. As Gornick (1986) suggests:

> If masculinity is predicated on a repudiation of the closeness and comforts offered by the original symbiosis and identification with the mother, then entering into a nonsexual intimacy with a woman therapist or analyst might lead those men with weaker defenses to feel overwhelmed and those men with stronger defenses to feel a greater need for vigilance. (p. 269)

Since men avail themselves of psychotherapy far less than women, the increasing likelihood of being matched with a female practitioner may make the therapeutic encounter appear even more menacing to the prospective male client. For these men, writes Gornick (1986), "seeing a woman as a therapist can be doubly shaming—the shame of being a patient as well as the shame of being in a subordinate position to a woman" (p. 270).[2] This potential experience of shame for men may be recognized on some level by therapists, as a recent study of referral patterns among psychoanalysts indicates that both male and female analysts overwhelmingly refer male patients to male therapists rather than their female colleagues (Mayer & de Marneffe, 1992). Therefore, as the feminization of psychotherapy continues and the possibility of working with a male therapist decreases, will men be even more reluctant to seek out psychotherapy as it is increasingly perceived as an endeavor constructed by and for women?

In this growing world without men, it is possible to imagine how males could be conceptualized as the "other"—the abuser, the distant and longed-for father, the savior, the unattainable lover or boyfriend, the molestor, the man who left one's mother pregnant and without support, the mythical but never realized means of attaining separateness, freedom, power. As adult men become more removed from family life in actuality, they become more subject to their children's unconscious fantasy life, untempered by reality. Since the hallmark of loss is both idealization and denigration, what a man is in reality can remain clouded in a labyrinth of self-blame, longing, and rage. Media myths and social stereotypes surrounding male icons and authority figures can loom large in fantasy lives unbounded by quotidian exposure to actual adult men. In her study of "Man-hating and Ambivalence in Women's Lives," Judith Levine (1992) reports that:

---

[2]It is interesting to witness how this shame is managed in film. From Alfred Hitchcock's *Spellbound* (1945) to Barbra Streisand's *The Prince of Tides* (1991), men are able to reverse their subordinate relationship to a female therapist through an overwhelming erotic power that compels the woman psychiatrist to transgress the boundaries of her professional role and devote both her professional and personal life to the cure of this one man. Through effecting her sexual and emotional surrender, the man effectively redresses the previously "shameful" power relationship that placed him in a subordinate position to a woman in authority.

Man-hating is born in the predominant quality of modern Western fatherhood: absence. . . .

The patriarchy's idealization of the father, and men generally; the girl's exclusion from the spoils of masculinity, its privilege, authority and agency; her hunger for the father himself, a figure who becomes ever more desirable as he recedes into the distance; the mother's simultaneous propping up and tearing down of the mythic all-powerful, perfect father—these social facts and personal feelings are arrayed around man-hating and ambivalence not in dot-to-dot lines of causality, but in a cluster of concurrences and contradictions. (pp. 186, 187)[3]

As psychotherapy becomes a women's field, the idea is reinforced that men are not or cannot be the ones to whom one turns for attention, empathy, or understanding. Just as women represented the "other" in the Freudian paradigm—based in the patriarchal family of late 19th century Vienna, built upon the authority of the oedipal father, and practiced largely by men—so now men may be approaching this status within the relational model—based in the declining authority and involvement of the father, built upon the deterministic influence of the mother, and practiced largely by women.

As we approach the 21st century, we need to be fully aware of all the implications that ensue when any part of our social world becomes the property of one sex alone. As a number of occupations have undergone feminization, we need to be particularly attentive to how that process not only affects economic and status variables but also how it affects the character of work itself, relations between the sexes, and our social life in general. As one of the premier helping professions, psychotherapy can have a tremendous influence on

---

[3]That "man-hating" may be on the increase is suggested by a recent poll. In 1990, the Roper Organization queried 3,000 women nationwide on their attitudes toward men, asking questions that had been part of an identical survey in 1970. In the poll conducted 20 years earlier, 66% of the women agreed with the statement that "most men are basically kind, gentle and thoughtful." In 1990, only 50% agreed, and 42% of those polled went even further, agreeing with the statement that men are "basically selfish and self-centered" ("Women Call Men Lazy," 1990, p. A-1).

people and on how we experience ourselves, others, and the world around us. It is second only to the family in terms of the power it can have in shaping the emotional lives of those who elect to partake of the process. The fact that men are no longer choosing this work, just as they are absenting themselves increasingly from families, suggests that responsiblity for tending to emotional concerns, psychological problems, and people's inner core of experience will fall even more into the hands of women.

This process portends a greater bifurcation in our social lives along gender lines. The traditional division of labor associated with men's identification with the public sphere and women's with the private has been eroded to some degree by women's greater labor force participation since World War II. Nonetheless, whatever erosion has occurred has taken place against the backdrop of a labor force segregated on the basis of gender. And this segregation continues to fall along predictable lines: Women numerically dominate occupations that can be seen as extensions of their traditional roles within the family. Nursing, social work, waitressing, school teaching, and day care, to name only a few, continue to be bastions of female employment. The new addition of psychotherapy to this litany robs society of an institution in which men traditionally have involved themselves in emotion work, in tolerating and immersing themselves in the intimate and messy problems real people experience on a day-to-day basis. Men's abandonment of the field of psychotherapy confirms the idea, nurtured in families, that if one is hurting inside, if one is depressed or anxious, it is women's job to fix it.

Toward an Ethic of Care in an Age of "Self-Sufficiency"

There are 30 to 40 million people without health care in this country. If we're going to bring it to the masses, it will be in the form of managed care. Granted, it won't be the Chippendale of psychotherapy—more likely it will be Levitz—but, how many people have ever been able to afford Chippendale?"

—*Nicholas Cummings*[1]

In what seems like the distant past, there was a vision in this country that valued mental health care and sought to make it available to people from all social classes and walks of life. It offered "the open warmth of community concern and capability" as the means of achieving "prevention, treatment and rehabilitation" of mental illness (Kennedy, 1963). Such a vision resonated with people's sense of the future, their sense of possibility. Through reform, scientific progress, and American know-how, social problems, such as mental illness, could be eradicated. In a 1962 *Look* magazine forum on what America would look like in 25 years, an assemblage of scholars, scientists, and politicians agreed that there would still be problems, such as "pockets of poverty" that needed to be ame-

[1]Founder of the largest freestanding professional school of psychology and the fastest growing managed health care company in the United States (quoted in Wylie, 1992c, p. 36).

liorated, but significant social change—"the kind that is painful and agonizing and that forces individuals and generations into a sense of radical disjuntion between traditional ways and contemporary realities—would henceforth be confined to developing nations, like Tunisia" (quoted in Skolnick, 1991, p. 2).

While such belief undoubtedly seems quaint from today's vantage point, the chasm that separates Americans in the 1990s from the hopefulness that pervaded this country in the early 1960s is also nothing less than tragic. Thirty years ago we cherished the belief that with time everyone would have the potential to take advantage of the "Chippendale" of life's necessities—from public education to secure employment to health care and social security in old age. This belief lies moribund today, as homelessness, high rates of unemployment, crime, a ravaged public school system, widespread environmental destruction, and a pervasive sense of despair about the future haunt our society. In this post-Watergate, post-Reagan era of cynicism, scarcity, and insecurity, "Levitz" seems about the best we can hope for, a realistic approach in an age when compromise and making do are our highest aims.

That mental health care seemingly has dropped to the bottom of our social priorities as a nation is unsurprising given the desperate fight local and state governments are waging to find resources to pay for the necessities of life—police and fire services, education, health care for the indigent, and infrastructure repair and maintenance. Certainly in this climate, professional attention to one's emotional and psychological needs can be seen as a luxury, something that the upper classes can afford but that everyone else can do without. If one's problems can be addressed, however, with a pill or six sessions of psychotherapy, then private insurance companies or perhaps even the state will be willing to foot the bill. If chemical solutions don't work, or if it is difficult to express oneself or trust a stranger enough to talk about intimate details of life in six sessions, then the burden of care reverts to the individual.

Throughout this book, I have tried to locate and describe one aspect of this burden and how it has come to rest on women's shoulders. As I see it, among its many meanings, the feminization of psychotherapy is one more example of how the messiness of everyday existence is tended to by women—as always within the family, and now outside of it as well. Changing diapers for the young and bedpans for the elderly has always been women's work. As that work moved outside the home—to the child care center, hospital, and retirement home—women followed. Now as psychotherapy is simultaneously endangered by outside forces and reconceptualized as "replacement therapy" for early maternal failures, women are the ones who are increasingly responsible for its practice. To the list of diapers and bedpans can be added the emotional pain of everyday life to which women in the work force now tend. The nurse, the child care worker, the nursing home attendant, the waitress, the secretary—that is, the people who bandage our wounds, cuddle our children, listen to the elderly, serve our food, make our coffee and our memos—are now occupationally joined by the women who listen to our problems.

Certainly psychotherapy is more than this. It is a skill, an intellectual endeavor, a profession whose acquisition marks a significant advancement in large numbers of women's occupational lives. That so many women are earning advanced degrees in order to practice as psychotherapists is both a personal achievement and an achievement for women in society as a whole. Yet these facts cannot blind us to the perhaps unwelcomed reality that the profession women are entering is changing dramatically and diminishing in status.

"Mothering" in Mean Times

Women now starting careers as psychotherapists face numerous contradictions in their professional lives. At a time when the relational model is ascendant, as the "real relationship" between client and therapist is touted as prerequisite to therapeutic cure, managed care mandates a short-term model of treatment. Rather than encouraging intensity, dependency, and exploration of the transference, brief treatment by its very nature discourages clients from becoming dependent on either the therapeutic process or the therapist herself. Typically its goal is to return a client to his or her previous state of functioning, to quickly resolve a crisis, to educate, to recommend a client seek a biochemical solution, or to suggest he or she pursue long-term psychotherapy at his or her own expense.

That practitioners are increasingly reading clinical theory that describes their work as fundamentally relational but are having to engage in nonrelational therapies to satisfy the mandates of managed care is bound to engender some degree of conflict, disillusionment, or frustration. Unable to practice what is considered right, up to date, curative, and/or in the best interests of the client, a therapist cannot feel wholly good about her work and perhaps even about herself as a clinician. Clearly, theorists who extol the relational model do not consider the actual exigencies of clinical practice facing most practitioners, and particularly new practitioners, today. The material realities of the profession remain outside the theoretical constructs and thinking of present-day psychodynamic authors just as much as they remained of little interest to Freud and his contemporaries.

Simultaneously, managed care and its short-term therapy model lacks virtually any theoretical underpinnings. Having arisen as a response to solely economic concerns, the HMOs and PPOs hiring and contracting with individual clinicians today typically care only about cost containment. How therapists choose to work within their apportioned number of sessions and what theoretical frameworks they adhere to is largely their business. As long as clients do not complain and therapists do not exceed the boundaries of the time allotted to complete their work, the arbiters of managed care are content.

This set of factors often places the clinician in the position of having to make do, compromise what she is reading or has been taught with what is required of her. While the demands of managed care are obviously contradictory for the psychodynamic therapist, they are also so for the feminist family therapist and feminist clinicians in general, whom family therapist Betty Carter lauds for staying "relationship oriented" while "new models [were] becoming 'solution-oriented'" (see Chapter 4).

The apparent virtue of being "relationship oriented" can also be seen as conflicting with the increasing need to market oneself as a private practitioner, even for a part-time private practice. Although professional organizations and journals have been astonishingly slow to react to the changes taking place in clinical practice, entrepreneurs not only acknowledge these changes but deluge therapists regularly through advertising and direct mail promotional campaigns on how to cope with these changes through marketing. As the publisher of the *Mental Health Marketing Strategies* newsletter explains in a typical piece of direct mail literature:

> I recognized early on that Medicaid patients, patients on welfare—patients who couldn't afford my services—would never help me support my family. The secret to developing a good practice is to get full fee paying patients. . . .
>
> It's not something anyone teaches you in your professional courses. As a matter of fact—colleges teach you enough skills to get a job working for a governmental agency—that will pay you a poverty level salary. They refuse to teach you the skills you need to build a private practice.
>
> *The secret skill you need to learn to make it all work—is how to market. . . .*
>
> *You've got to learn the science of marketing.* You have to get your message heard by people—who still have private health insurance—or who have cash—and who need your service. (Budman, n.d.)

This sort of marketing ethic seems to depend on skills and attitudes toward one's work that stand in opposition to remothering and empathy. It reveres self-aggrandizement, treating potential clients as objects and shunning those on Medicaid, welfare, and even those who cannot pay a full fee, that is, those most in need. Its lingua franca is money. It celebrates those who can network, sell, manipulate, and exploit untapped markets of potential therapy consumers. And if it promotes any form of empathy, it is empathy for the wealthy or well insured alone.

Therefore, not only does the primacy placed on marketing in many ways contravene the values and emphases of the relational model, it suggests what kind of clinician may best succeed in the increasingly crowded and competitive arena of private practice. Those who think only of what is in the best interest of their clients, who wish to treat people from diverse backgrounds and with diverse needs, and who neglect self-promotion, networking, and strategizing about potential markets for their services will not prosper as private practitioners. They will be the ones who of necessity link up with managed care, or who will be compelled to find means of supporting themselves outside the provision of direct clinical services.

It is often the case that women do not find marketing and self-promotion easily acquired skills. Their reasons for becoming psychotherapists (and also those of many men) often have little to do with running a small business, which is what private practice often resembles—particularly in increasingly saturated markets that demand aggressive self-promotion. Women typically set lower fees and have lower incomes than their male colleages, as a 1992 survey by *Psychotherapy Finances* (Vol. 17, No. 12) demonstrated. Among the almost 2,000 full-time private practitioners polled, female clinical psychologists at the doctoral level had a median income of $62,500, whereas males had one of $81,818. At the master's level, women earned $47,000 and men $61,538. And for social workers, women averaged $47,000, and their male counterparts $57,273. While this survey does not seem to have taken into account how long each clinician had been practicing—a variable that might mitigate this differential—it is generally recognized that women, and particularly those new to the field, have more difficulty promoting themselves and demanding the same fees as their male counterparts. As psychoanalyst Zeborah Schachtel (1986) points out:

> Male supervisees seem less stressed by boundary issues, such as management of fees and absences, probably because they feel less pulled by the gender experience of "giving and providing" than does the female, though each gender may also

try to fight the pull. . . . My impression from discussion with colleages and from supervision is that the management of the external boundary issues is particularly difficult and stressful for women and that those issues often are not managed well. (p. 250)

It seems entirely possible that in the future, private practice may become the domain of the successful entrepreneur, and that those who find the primacy of marketing and self-promotion objectionable or simply unattainable will be excluded from this form of professional pursuit. As Mary Sykes Wylie (1992c) suggests, "it is possible that, at least in private practice, the style and personality of the therapist—even the sort of person who is drawn to doing therapy in the first place—is rapidly shifting and adapting to a new, harsher economic climate" (p. 32). That the men who remain in the field may be better entrepreneurs and, therefore, represent a disproportionate share of well-paid private practitioners does not seem unlikely. They simply may have more of the attributes in general that closely resemble the "style and personality" needed in these harsher economic times. Today it is primarily the male psychotherapist who founds provider organizations for managed care, who sends out direct mail literature touting his marketing strategies, who offers seminars on how to earn large incomes from private practice, and who writes books and newsletters on how to triumph over the growing "therapist glut." This tendency thus suggests yet another bifurcation of the field of psychotherapy along gender lines, one that again may limit women's access to authority and power.

From Self-Sufficiency to an Ethic of Care[2]

The feminization of psychotherapy signifies a set of dual problems for women. On the one hand, it is intimately tied to the denigration of psychotherapy in our society in general—its

---

[2]My thinking on an ethic of care has been greatly influenced by the work of Joan Tronto (See Tronto [in press]).

deskilling and declassing, its displacement by the medical model, its decreasing value in the eyes of the state, employers, and managed care. Certainly, female clinicians' fate is tied to the fate of the field in which they practice. On the other hand, the potential for women to remain the primary care providers of mental health services in HMOs, PPOs, and extant community clinics, while the declining number of men in the field serve as its administrators, supervisors, entrepreneurs, theorists, and perhaps even its private practitioners, seems great. These dual foci suggest that the future of psychotherapy and the future of its growing body of female practitioners resides in how society chooses to value psychotherapy as a helping profession and how women within the profession are valued. If the majority of the field's members remain second class citizens despite their numerical strength, then certainly the status of the field itself is imperiled.

Some means of rectifying problems may be relatively attainable. First, there needs to be a general recognition in all of the psychotherapy professional groupings—but particularly in clinical psychology at both the master's and doctoral levels—that there is an oversupply of clinicians. Freestanding, tuition-driven professional schools cannot continue producing greater and greater numbers of graduates with literally no attention to the forces of supply and demand. Second, there needs to be greater attention to standards at all levels of graduate school—admissions, progressions, and graduation. The desire for maintaining the largest number of students, paying the highest tuitions the market will bear cannot be the criterion upon which graduate schools select, educate, and graduate students.

Further, these freestanding schools, which are increasingly responsible for the bulk of master's level and doctoral level psychotherapists, have a duty to educate students in the scholarly and theoretical histories and current debates of their field. Clinicians-in-training must be seen as having the potential to transcend mere technician or "journeyman" status and think of themselves as part of long-established intellectual traditions. As pointed out in Chapter 5, this is of particular importance for women, who so frequently do not feel authorized to speak and write theoretically.

Students also must be instructed in the occupational realities of psychotherapy practice. They cannot be trained according to the model of a full-time private practitioner who autonomously determines the course of treatment for her clients. The business aspects of psychotherapy practice cannot be either overlooked or disparaged but must be acknowledged and illuminated for new entrants to the field. If clinical practice is going to be conceptualized as a means of filling in the deficits arising out of the early mother–child relationship, then this conceptualization must be premised on an expansive vision of mothering, one that is not only empathic and nurturing but also fully engaged in the world, clear witted, and resourceful. With such a vision in mind, female practitioners should not only be able to adequately assess the exigencies of their field but actively choose, create, administer, and lead within it. Business considerations may seem outside the domain of a "professional," perhaps anathema to some, but the female clinician who eschews economics and the material underpinnings of her field will diminish her prospects and contribute to women's overall lack of power professionally.

In keeping with this perspective, it appears foolish to respond to the burgeoning managed care movement through outrage, belittling, or denial. For better or worse, it is the future, and it is only in the female practitioner's interest to not merely understand it but look for ways that she can help construct and mold it. While such a goal may appear to be out of reach for the average clinician, managed mental health care delivery is in a state of growth and invention; its parameters have not been set nor its procedures and modalities codified. Currently, there are innovators in the field who have established cost-effective managed care organizations that promote clinical decision making rather than case management.[3] Such a model allows the clinician and her face-to-face clinical supervisor to determine the course of therapy, rather than a case manager who sits at a distance, or worse yet, a

[3]The founders of Pacific Applied Psychology Associates in Berkeley, California, Gregory Alter and Neil Dickman, represent one such example.

computerized decision tree—something increasingly employed by case management firms. While such innovation is constrained by the demands of cost containment, there is room for allowing practitioners greater (and lesser) degrees of autonomy and control over the work process. And women can only profit by finding ways to insert themselves in the creation and definition of managed care.

Such high demands of the female psychotherapist do not mean to suggest that it is she alone who holds the solutions to the dilemmas facing her and her rapidly feminizing occupation. I clearly believe that the manner in which female family therapists have approached the power structure within family therapy and have organized themselves to ensure women's visibility at all levels of their profession can serve as a model throughout the field of psychotherapy. But a far greater effort and transformation needs to occur for psychotherapy in general and its female practitioners in particular to garner authority, status, and significant levels of recompense in the United States today.

As long as our society denigrates an ethic of care and celebrates self-sufficiency, autonomy, and rigorous competitiveness as its highest virtues—the very emblems of what it means to be an American—women and their occupational choices will lose out, consigned to afterthought and oversight. Just as women's work within the home has traditionally been taken for granted, so too their employment in the public domain can be undervalued and poorly compensated. Early childhood education, school teaching, nursing, and librarianship are all examples of women's work that is accorded little status relative to the education and skill levels required. Caring for the young, the sick, or the needy remains outside our long-standing national obsession with the vigorous pursuit of self-interest. As a country, the United States does not have an impressive history of caring for its needy, less self-sufficient citizens relative to similarly developed nations. But in the current political atmosphere of denouncing "big government," new taxes, and "welfare cheats," we are moving even further away from making aid, support, and guidance of our citizenry a national priority. We are increasingly a country where aid and nurturance are meted out haphazardly, in piecemeal fashion, with little social value attached—and typically provided by women.

In such an environment, psychotherapy—like all "helping professions"—cannot thrive or prevail. Its very premises of ameliorating psychic pain and promoting emotional growth through some form of sustained and caring relationship stand outside our renewed social reverence for self-sufficiency. The medical model facilitates this veneration through its promotion of chemical solutions that circumvent reliance on other human beings for help. Requiring medication is not seen as a virtue, but it is an acceptable form of self-preservation in an age that prefers to see almost all forms of psychopathology—from alcoholism to schizophrenia—as disease processes rather than as problems that may require long-term forms of care that foster any form of dependency.

To be dependent in our society is to not be fully human, not fully capable of participating in the social arena. Dependence is the concern of domesticity or the undervalued and underfunded corners of public life. If it extends beyond childhood, it is relegated to the recesses and shadows of society, where it is largely women who attend and minister. As we move to the close of the 20th century, it appears that psychotherapy as an occupation is moving further into those recesses and shadows. Its endurance and advancement, and that of its female practitioners, ultimately cannot be understood nor truly fostered outside of what we as a nation choose to value and accord recognition. The feminizing field of psychotherapy and the women within it can only begin to gain authority and respect for their work when our society can move toward sanctioning an ethic of care for its citizens and viewing dependency as a normal part of human existence that occurs throughout the life course.

References

Albee, G. W. (1959). *Mental health manpower trends.* New York: Basic Books.

Alexander, F., & French, T. M. (1946). *Psychoanalytic therapy: Principles and application.* New York: Ronald Press.

Almeida, R., & Silvestri, K. (1992). Letters to the editor. *Family Therapy Networker, 16,* 8.

Atwood, G., & Stolorow, R. (1984). *Structures of subjectivity.* Hillsdale, N.J.: Analytic Press.

Auerbach, N. (1981). Maji and maidens: The romance of the Victorian Freud. *Critical Inquiry, 8.*

Baruch, E. H., & Serrano, L. J. (1988). *Women analyze women.* New York: New York University Press.

Benjamin, J. (1988). *The bonds of love.* New York: Pantheon.

Bernard, J. (1981). The good-provider role: Its rise and fall. *American Psychologist, 36*(1), 1–12.

Berube, A. (1990). Coming out under fire. New York: Free Press.

Bourne, P. G., & Wikler, N. J. (1982). Commitment and the cultural mandate: Women in medicine. In R. Kahn-Hut, A. Kaplan Daniels, & R. Colvard (Eds.), *Women and work* (pp. 111–122). New York: Oxford University Press.

Braude, M. (1987). Women psychiatrists change the American Psychiatric Association. In M. Braude (Ed.), *Women, power, and therapy: Issues for women* (pp. 183–186). New York: Haworth Press.

Braverman, H. (1974). *Labor and monopoly capital.* New York: Monthly Review Press.

Brown, C. (1987). Consumption norms, work roles, and economic growth, 1918–80. In C. Brown & J. A. Pechman (Eds.), *Gender in the workplace* (pp. 13–58). Washington, DC: The Brookings Institution.

Buckhout, R. (Ed.). (1971). Toward social change: A handbook for those who will. New York: Harper & Row.

Buntman, P. Four secrets of building a $10,000–15,000—even a $20,000 a month private practice [Direct mail literature]. *Mental Health Marketing Strategies.*

Capshew, J. H., & Laszlo, A.C. (1986). "We would not take no for an answer": Women psychologists and gender politics during World War II. *Journal of Social Issues, 42*(1), 157–180.

Carter, B. (1992). Stonewalling feminism. *The Family Therapy Networker, 16*(1), 64–69.

Carter, M. J., & Carter, S. B. (1981). Women's recent progress in the professions, or women get a ticket to ride after the gravy train has left the station. *Feminist Studies, 7*(3), 477–504.

Chodorow, N. (1978). *The reproduction of mothering.* Berkeley: University of California Press.

Chodorow, N. (1989). *Feminism and psychoanalytic theory.* New Haven: Yale University Press.

Chodorow, N. (1991). Where have all the eminent women psychoanalysts gone. In J. Blau & N. Goodman (Eds.), *Social roles and social institutions.* Boulder, CO: Westview Press.

Chodorow, N., & Contratto, S. (1990). The fantasy of the perfect mother. In N. Chodorow, *Feminism and psychoanalytic theory.* New Haven: Yale University Press.

Cooper, A. (1990). The future of psychoanalysis: Challenges and opportunities. *The Psychoanalytic Quarterly, 59,* 177–196.

Coyne, J. (1992). Letters to the editor. *Family Therapy Networker, 16,* 7.

Cummings, N. A. (1977). Professional schools in psychology. *International encylopedia of psychiatry, psychology, psychoanalysis and neurology.*

Cummings, N. A. (1986). The dismantling of our health system: Strategies for the survival of psychological practice. *American Psychologist, 41,* 426–431.

Currie, E., Dunn, R., & Fogarty, D. (1990). The fading dream: Economic crisis and the new inequality. In K. V. Hansen & I. J. Philipson (Eds.), *Women, class and the feminist imagination* (pp. 319–337). Philadelphia: Temple University Press.

Davies, M. W. (1982). *Women's place is at the typewriter: Office work and office workers, 1870–1930.* Philadelphia: Temple University Press.

De Titta, M., Robinowitz, M. D., & More, W. W. (1991). The future of psychiatry: Psychiatrists of the future. *American Journal of Psychiatry, 148*(7), 853–858.

Doctors of desire. (1991, August 4). *San Francisco Chronicle*, p. A-18.

Dorken, H., & Bennett, B. E. (1986). How professional psychology can shape its future. In H. Dorken (Ed.), *Professional psychology in transition*. San Francisco: Jossey-Bass.

Dorken, H., & VandenBos, G. R. (1986). Characteristics of 20,000 patients and their psychologists. In H. Dorken (Ed.), *Professional psychology in transition* (pp. 20–37). San Francisco: Jossey-Bass.

Dougherty, D. (1988). Children's mental health problems and services: Current federal efforts and policy implications. *American Psychologist, 43*, 808–811.

Ehrenreich, B. (1983). *The hearts of men*. Garden City, NY: Anchor Press.

Ehrenreich, B. (1989). *Fear of falling*. New York: Harper Perennial.

Elmer-Dewitt, P. (1992, July 6). Depression: The growing role of drug therapies. *Time*, pp. 57–60.

Fox, R. E., Kovacs, A.L., & Graham, S. R. (1985). Proposals for a revolution in the preparation and regulation of professional psychologists. *American Psychologist, 40*(9), 1042–1049.

Freud, S. (1912). The dynamics of transference. In J. Strachey (Ed. & Trans.), *The standard edition of the complete psychological works of Sigmund Freud* (Vol. 20). London: Hogarth Press. (Original work published 1959)

Friedman, L. J. (1990). *Menninger: The family and the clinic*. New York: Alfred Knopf.

Fromm-Reichmann, F. (1950). *Principles of intensive psychotherapy*. Chicago: University of Chicago Press.

Furstenberg, F. F. (1988). Good dads–bad dads: Two faces of fatherhood. In A. Cherlin (Ed.), *The changing American family and public policy* (pp. 193–218). Washington, DC: The Urban Institute Press.

Furstenberg, F. F., & Cherlin, A. (1991). *Divided families: What happens to children when parents part*. Cambridge, MA: Harvard University Press.

Furstenberg, F. F., & Mullan Harris, K. (1990). *The disappearing American father? Divorce and the waning significance of biological parenthood*. Unpublished manuscript, University of Pennsylvania, Department of Sociology, Philadelphia.

Gardiner, J. K. (1992). Psychoanalysis and feminism: An American humanist's view. *Signs, 17*(2), 437–454.

Garrison, J. (1991, December 8). Employers shrink from therapy bills. *San Francisco Examiner*.

Gill, M. M. (1954). Psychoanalysis and exploratory psychotherapy. *Journal of the American Psychoanalytic Association, 2,* 771–797.

Gill, M. M. (1984). Psychoanalysis and psychotherapy: A revision. *International Review of Psycho-Analysis, 11,* 161–179.

Gilligan, C. (1982). *In a different voice.* Cambridge, MA: Harvard University Press.

Goldberg, A. (1990). *The prison house of psychoanalysis.* Hillsdale, NJ: Analytic Press.

Goldberger, M., & Evans, D. (1985). On transference manifestations in male patients with female analysts. *International Journal of Psycho-Analysis, 66,* 295–309.

Goleman, D. (1990, May 17). New paths to mental health put strains on some healers. *New York Times,* pp. 1, B-7.

Golding, J., Lang, K., Eymard, L., & Shadish, W. (1988). The buck stops here: A survey of the financial status of Ph.D. graduate students in psychology, 1966–1987. *American Psychologist, 43*(12).

Goodrich, T. (1991). Women and power: Perspectives for family therapy. New York: Norton.

Goodrich, T., Rampage, C., & Ellman, B. (1988). *Feminist family therapy: A casebook.* New York: Norton.

Gornick, L. (1986). Developing a new narrative: The woman therapist and the male patient. In J. Alpert (Ed.), *Psychoanalysis and women: Contemporary reappraisals.* Hillsdale, NJ: Analytic Press.

Green, R. (1990). Family therapy training: The rising tide of mediocrity. *American Family Therapy Association Newsletter, 40,* 3–8.

Guntrip, H. (1971). *Psychoanalytic theory, therapy and the self.* New York: Basic Books.

Hale, N. G. (1978). From Berggasse XIX to Central Park West: The Americanization of psychoanalysis, 1919–1940. *Journal of the History of the Behavioral Sciences, 14,* 299–315.

Hendrix, K. (1992, April 19). When women turn to matters of the mind. *Los Angeles Times.*

Hilgard, E. (1987). *Psychology in America: A historical survey.* New York: Harcourt Brace Jovanovich.

Hochschild, A. R. (1983). *The managed heart.* Berkeley: University of California Press.

Hoffer, A. (1991). The Freud-Ferenczi controversy—a living legacy. *International Review of Psycho-Analysis, 18,* 465–472.

Holroyd, J. C., & Brodsky, A. M. (1977). Psychologists' attitudes and practices regarding erotic and nonerotic physical contact with patients. *American Psychologist, 32*(10), 843–849.

Howard, A., Pion, G. M., Gottfredson, G. D., Flattau, P. E., Oskamp, S., Pfafflin, S. M., Bray, D. W., & Burstein, A. G. (1986). The Changing Face of American Psychology. *American Psychologist, 41*(12), 1311–1327.

Jacobs, J. A. (1989). *Revolving doors: Sex segregation and women's careers.* Stanford, CA: Stanford University Press.

Jenson, J., Hagen, E., & Reddy, C. (Eds.). (1988). *Feminization of the labor force.* New York: Oxford University Press.

Jones, E. E., & Zoppel, C. L. (1982). Impact of client and therapist gender on psychotherapy process and outcome. *Journal of Consulting and Clinical Psychology, 50*(2), 259–272.

Kaplan, A. G. (1987). Reflections on gender and psychotherapy. In M. Braude (Ed.), *Women, Power, and Therapy, Issues for Women* (pp. 11–24). New York: The Haworth Press.

Kenkel, M. B. (1991, February). The feminization of psychology. Paper presented at the meeting of the National Council of Schools of Professional Psychology, Tucson, AZ.

Kennedy, J. F. (1963, February 5). Special message to the Congress on mental illness and mental retardation. (Quoted in Buckhout, 1971, p. 375.)

Kiesler, C. A. (1982). Public and professional myths about mental hospitalization: An empirical reassessment of policy-related beliefs. *American Psychologist, 37.*

Kiesler, C. A., & Morton, T. L. (1988). Psychology and public policy in the health care revolution. *American Psychologist, 43.*

Kirshner, L. A ., Genack, A., & Hauser, S. T. (1978). Effects of gender on short-term psychotherapy. *Psychotherapy: Theory, Research and Practice,* 15(2).

Klerman, G. L. (1983). The efficacy of psychotherapy as the basis for public policy. *American Psychologist, 38,* 929–934.

Kohut, H. (1971). *The analysis of the self.* New York: International Universities Press.

Kohut, H. (1977). *The restoration of the self.* New York: International Universities Press.

Kohout, J. (1991). *Changes in supply: Women in psychology.* Paper presented at the meeting of the American Psychological Association, San Francisco, CA.

Korn, J. H. (1984). New odds on acceptance into Ph.D. programs in psychology. *American Psychologist, 39*(2), 179–180.

Levine, J. (1992). *My enemy, my love: Man-hating and ambivalence in women's lives.* New York: Doubleday.

Levine, M. (1981). *The history and politics of community mental health*. New York: Oxford University Press.

Lubove, R. (1971). *The professional altruist: The emergence of social work as a career 1880–1930*. Cambridge, MA: Harvard University Press.

Marshall, J. (1992). Single parents struggle with poverty. *San Francisco Chronicle*, 6/11/92, p. A-14.

Mayer, E. L., & de Marneffe, D. (1992). When theory and practice diverge: Gender-related patterns of referral to psychoanalysts. *Journal of the American Psychoanalytic Association, 40*(2), 551–585.

Menninger, W. C. (1967). Psychiatry and the war. In W. C. Menninger (Ed.), *A psychiatrist for a troubled world*. New York: Viking Press.

Menninger, W. C. (1967). Psychiatric experience in the war, 1941–1946. In W. C. Menninger (Ed.), *A psychiatrist for a troubled world*. New York: Viking Press.

Miller, J. B. (1976). *Toward a new psychology of women*. Boston: Beacon Press.

Mitchell, S. (1988). *Relational concepts in psychoanalysis: An integration*. Cambridge, MA: Harvard University Press.

Modell, A. (1984). *Psychoanalysis in a new context*. New York: International University Press.

Mogul, K. M. (1982). Overview: The sex of the therapist. *The American Journal of Psychiatry, 139*(1), 1–11.

Never-Married women and child support. (1990, August 27). *San Francisco Chronicle*.

NIMH landmark study. (1990, October 12). *San Francisco Chronicle*.

O'Connell, A. N., & Russo, N. F. (Eds.). (1983). Models of achievement: Reflections of eminent women in psychology. New York: Columbia University Press.

Ogden, T. (1989). *The primitive edge of experience*. Northvale, NJ: Jason Aronson.

Orlinsky, D. E., & Howard, K. I. (1976). The effects of sex of therapist on the theraputic experiences of women. *Psychotherapy: Theory, Research, and Practice, 13*(1), 82–88.

Ostertag, P. A., & McNamara, J. R. (1991). "Feminization" of psychology. *Psychology of Women Quarterly, 15*, 349–369.

Peterson, D. R. (1985). Twenty years of practitioner training in psychology. *American Psychologist, 40*(4), 441–451.

Pittman, F. (1992). It's not my fault. *The Family Therapy Networker, 16*(1), 56–63.

Reisman, J. M. (1976). *A history of clinical psychology*. New York: Irvington Publishers.

Reskin, B. F. (1990). Culture, commerce, and gender: The feminization of book editing. In B. F. Reskin & P. A. Roos (Eds.), *Job queues, gender queues* (pp. 93–110). Philadelphia: Temple University Press.

Reskin, B. F., & Roos, P. A. (1990). *Job queues, gender queues.* Philadelphia: Temple University Press.

Reskin, B. F., & Hartmann, H. I. (1986). *Women's work, men's work: Sex segregation on the job.* Washington, DC: National Academy Press.

Robiner, W. N. (1991). How many psychologists are needed? A call for a national psychology human resource agenda. *Professional Psychology: Research and Practice, 22*(6), 427–440.

Roos, P. (1985). *Gender and work: A comparative analysis of industrial societies.* Albany, NY: SUNY Press.

Rothman, S. (1978). *Woman's proper place: A history of changing ideals and practices, 1870 to the Present.* New York: Basic Books.

Ruddick, S. (1990). Thinking about fathers. In M. Hirsch & E. Fox Keller (Eds.), *Conflicts in feminism.* New York: Routledge.

Sayers, J. (1990). *Mothering psychoanalysis.* London: Hamish Hamilton.

Schachtel, Z. (1986). The "impossible profession" considered from a gender perspective. In J. Alpert (Ed.), *Psychoanalysis and women: Contemporary reappraisals.* Hillsdale, NJ: Analytic Press.

Scull, A. (1977). *Decarceration: Community treatment and the deviant.* Englewood Cliffs, NJ: Prentice-Hall.

Seeley, J. R. (1961, January). The Americanization of the unconscious. *The Atlantic.*

Shackelford, M. (1991). *A question of authority.* Unpublished paper, New York University Postdoctoral Psychology Program in Psychotherapy and Psychoanalysis, New York.

Simon, R. (1992). Editorial. *Family Therapy Networker, 16,* 2.

Skolnick, A. (1991). *Embattled paradise.* New York: Basic Books.

Skolnikoff, A. Z. (1981). *The activation of different conflicts in depressed women with male and female therapists.* Unpublished manuscript, San Francisco Psychoanalytic Institute.

The squeeze on psychoanalytic chains. (1991, October 26). *New York Times,* p. 29.

Stoller, R. (1974). Facts and fancies: An examination of Freud's concept of bisexuality. In J. Strouse (Ed.), *Women and analysis.* New York: Grossman Publishers.

Strober, M. H., & Arnold, C. L. (1987). The dynamics of occupational segregation among bank tellers. In C. Brown & J. A.

Pechman (Eds.), *Gender in the workplace* (pp. 107–148). Washington, DC: The Brookings Institution.

Survey finds fewer blacks, men in teaching. (1992, July 7). *San Francisco Chronicle.*

Taube, C. A., Burns, B. J., & Kessler, L. (1984). Patients of psychiatrists and psychologists in office-based practice: 1980. *American Psychologist, 39,* 1435–1446.

Touhey, J. C. (1974). Effects of additional women professionals on ratings of occupational prestige and desirability. *Journal of Personality and Social Psychology, 29,* 86–89.

The way we were. (1992). *Family Therapy Networker, 16,* 30–49.

Tronto, J. (in press). Moral boundaries: Political argument for an ethic of care. New York: Routledge.

Wallerstein, R. S. (1989). Psychoanalysis and psychotherapy: An historical perspective. *International Journal of Psycho-Analysis, 70,* 563–591.

Whitehead, B. D. (1993, April). Dan Quayle was right. *The Atlantic,* pp. 47–84.

Williams, C. (1989). *Gender differences at work: Women and men in nontraditional work.* Berkeley: University of California Press.

Winnicott, D. W. (1958). *Through paediatrics to psycho-analysis.* London: The Hogarth Press.

Winnicott, D. W. (1965). *The maturational process and the facilitating environment.* New York: International Universities Press.

Women call men lazy, self-centered. (1990, April 28). *San Francisco Examiner,* p. A-1.

Wylie, M. S. (1992a). The evolution of a revolution. *The Family Therapy Networker, 16*(1), 16–29.

Wylie, M. S. (1992b). Toeing the bottom line. *The Family Therapy Networker, 16*(2), 30–75.

Wylie, M. S. (1992c). Revising the dream. *The Family Therapy Networker, 16*(4), 10–23.

Zimet, C. N. (1989). The mental health care revolution: Will psychology survive? *American Psychologist, 44,* 703–708.

Index

n indicates that entry will be found in a footnote